D0301962

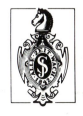

W. J. MacLennan · N. R. Peden

Metabolic and Endocrine Problems in the Elderly

With 29 Figures

Springer-Verlag
London Berlin Heidelberg New York
Paris Tokyo

W. J. MacLennan, MD, FRCP (Glas., Ed., Lond.)
Professor of Geriatric Medicine, University of Edinburgh, Edinburgh
EH10 5SB, Scotland, UK

N. R. Peden, MA, MB, FRCP(Ed.)
Consultant Physician and Endocrinologist, Falkirk and District Royal
Infirmary, Major's Loan, Falkirk FK1 5QE, Scotland, UK

ISBN 3–540–19541–6 Springer-Verlag Berlin Heidelberg New York
ISBN 0–387–19541–6 Springer-Verlag New York Berlin Heidelberg

British Library Cataloguing in Publication Data
MacLennan, W. J.
Metabolic and endocrine problems in the elderly.
1. Man. Endocrine system. Diseases   2. Old persons. Metabolic disorders & nutritional
disorders   I. Title   II. Peden, N. R.   616.4
ISBN 3–540–19541–6

Library of Congress Cataloging-in-Publication Data
MacLennan, W. J.
Metabolic and endocrine problems in the elderly/W. J. MacLennan, N. R. Peden.
p. cm.   Includes index.
ISBN 0–387–19541–6 (U.S.)   1. Endocrine glands—Diseases—Age factors.
2. Metabolism—Disorders—Age factors.   3. Aged—Diseases.   I. Peden, N. R.,
1950–   . II. Title.
[DNLM: 1. Endocrine Diseases—in old age.   2. Metabolic Diseases—in old age.
WK 100 M164m]   RC649.M33   1989   618.97'64—dc19   88-38512

© Springer-Verlag Berlin Heidelberg 1989
Printed in Great Britain

The use of registered names, trademarks etc. in this publication does not imply, even in the
absence of a specific statement, that such names are exempt from the relevant laws and
regulations and therefore free for general use.

Product Liability: The publisher can give no guarantee for information about drug dosage and
application thereof contained in this book. In every individual case the respective user must
check its accuracy by consulting other pharmaceutical literature.

Filmset by Tradeset Photosetting Ltd, Welwyn Garden City, UK
Printed by The Alden Press, Osney Mead, Oxford, UK

2128/3916–543210 (Printed on acid-free paper)

Preface

Illness in old age is characterised by vague and atypical presenting features which are often missed and wrongly attributed to the ageing process. This is particularly true of endocrine disorders where hypothyroidism may masquerade as dementia, where electrolyte imbalance may cause lassitude, and where diabetes mellitus may produce a wide range of complications commonly associated with ageing. It is our intention that our book provide straightforward practical guidance in this difficult area by delineating the effects of ageing on endocrine function and the clinical consequences of these; and by describing in detail the wide range of presenting clinical features of endocrine disease in the elderly.

Physicians are also often baffled and misled by the effects of ageing and disease on laboratory tests used in the investigation of endocrine disease. Our book describes these changes in detail, and gives guidance on which tests are most appropriate. Ageing and disease also produce subtle changes in the response of patients to drugs and replacement, and this is also discussed in detail.

Subjects included separately and in depth include thyroid disease, the clinical features and treatment of diabetes, postmenopausal changes, bone disease, fluid and electrolyte imbalance, energy imbalance, and drugs causing endocrine and metabolic disorders. These have been chosen because we consider that they present problems which are particularly relevant to the elderly. Many other issues are covered in general textbooks of endocrinology and have been omitted.

Several excellent accounts of the endocrinology of ageing are available in the literature. Most, however, have concentrated on reviewing in depth a few selected topics. While therefore they are invaluable as sources of background information, they are of less use to the clinician in his management of everyday problems. We hope that our simple and didactic account will serve this purpose.

July 1988   W.J.MacL.
                                                                         N.R.P.

Contents

1 Ageing and Endocrine Function

An understanding of the effects which ageing has on endocrine function is fundamental to the correct interpretation of the clinical and biochemical features of endocrine disease in old age. In some instances, as in hyperthyroidism, ageing modifies the physical signs. In others, as in carbohydrate metabolism, ageing changes the reference values, so that there is the semantic problem of whether values which are common are also normal.

A phenomenon less frequently appreciated is that in addition to changing norms, ageing also increases variation. Any description of ageing and endocrine function which fails to take this into account is an oversimplification.

Hypothalamo-pituitary Function

Ageing is associated with a decline in the hypothalamic concentrations of neurotransmitters, including catecholamines, γ-amino-butyric acid and acetylcholine (Everitt 1980). Coupled with this, there is a decline in the sensitivity of the hypothalamus to changing concentrations of some hormones and metabolites. An example is that the threshold of the hypothalamic appetite centre to the inhibitory effect of glucose is often elevated in old age (Dilman 1976). Again, corticosteroids are less effective in suppressing hypothalamic activity in the elderly. The extent to which this influences anterior pituitary function varies with the hormone involved.

Growth Hormone

Recent studies have shown a decrease in the nocturnal secretion of growth hormone particularly during the first 3 h of sleep in elderly as compared with young men (Prinz et al. 1983) and similar observations have been made in Rhesus monkeys (Kaler et al. 1986). Serum somatomedin levels also diminish in old age (Pavlov et al. 1986) and correlate with diminished growth hormone levels (Florini et al.

1985). Again, though growth hormone responses to hyperglycaemia are unaffected by age, men over 40 years of age show reduced growth hormone responses to growth hormone releasing hormone (GHRH) (Shibasaki et al. 1984) and a negative correlation between age and growth hormone responsiveness to GHRH has been shown in men and women, with circulating oestradiol concentrations having a significant effect on responses in women (Lang et al. 1987). This raises the possibility that a proportion of elderly subjects are growth hormone deficient with resulting effects on bone and muscle mass.

Thyroid-Stimulating Hormone (TSH)

Around one in ten men and one in four women over the age of 60 have high serum concentrations of TSH (Table 1.1) (Sawin et al. 1979). These levels are rarely associated with low thyroxine levels in healthy old people, and few people with an isolated serum TSH elevation proceed to hypothyroidism.

Table 1.1. Percentages of men and women with elevated serum TSH levels (Sawin et al. 1979)

	Percentage with moderately elevated TSH >5 <10 mU/l	Percentage with markedly elevated TSH >10 mU/l
Men	8.2	2.7
Women	16.9	7.1

In healthy old people, the standard dose of thyrotrophin releasing hormone (TRH) stimulates a normal increase in the serum TSH concentration while a post-mortem study has shown that the hypothalamic content of TRH does not change significantly with age (Ordene et al. 1983; Harman et al. 1984; Parker and Porter 1984).

Adreno-corticotrophic Hormone (ACTH) and Beta-endorphin

These anterior pituitary peptides are produced from a common precursor molecule, pro-opiomelanocortin and are secreted concomitantly (Imura 1985). The circadian rhythm of plasma ACTH and cortisol is not affected by age (Rolandi et al. 1987) but the circadian changes in beta-endorphin levels present in young individuals disappear in old age. The mechanism of this is unclear.

The response of ACTH to the stress of surgery is similar in young and elderly subjects (Arnetz et al. 1984).

Prolactin

In postmenopausal women there is a rise in plasma prolactin concentrations (Figure. 1.1) (Govoni et al. 1983). This itself is not of clinical importance, but

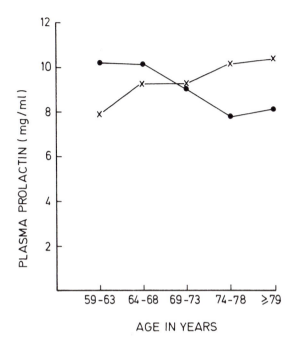

Fig. 1.1. Plasma prolactin level in elderly men (*circles*) and women (*crosses*). (After Govoni et al. 1983.)

probably reflects the decrease in pituitary inhibition which follows a reduction in hypophyseal dopaminergic activity. No such changes occur in men, but an inverse correlation has been reported between frequency of sexual intercourse and prolactin levels in the elderly (Weizmann and Hart 1983). The prolactin response to surgical stress is reduced in the elderly, particularly in older men (Arnetz et al. 1984).

Gonadotrophic Hormones in Men

Plasma levels of luteinising hormone (LH) and follicle stimulating hormone (FSH) are increased in elderly men (Muta et al. 1981; Deslypere and Vermeulen 1984).

Gonadotrophic Hormones in Women

After the menopause there is a threefold rise in plasma LH concentrations compared with a tenfold increase in those of FSH (Mills and Mahesh 1977). Following an initial postmenopausal rise in gonadotrophin concentrations, there is a progressive fall in these so that after 30 years they are at about half the maximal levels (Chakravarti et al. 1976). Surprisingly the gonadotrophin releasing hormone content of the hypothalamus is lower in elderly than premenopausal women (Parker and Porter 1984).

Pineal Gland

Plasma melatonin concentrations in the elderly are about half those found in young adults while at all ages, melatonin secretion increases at night and falls by day. Maximal levels in old people occur in October, whereas in the young these occur in January, suggesting an age related change in the hypothalamic control of secretion (Tointon et al. 1984). Histological studies have shown no change in the structure or function of pinealocytes.

Thyroid Gland

Though total serum thyroxine levels are unchanged there is a marginal reduction in serum total tri-iodothyronine levels (Caplan et al. 1981; Harman et al. 1984). This coupled with decreased degradation rates of thyroxine and tri-iodothyronine suggests an overall reduction in thyroid hormone production. The only clinical relevance of these changes is that, in establishing ranges of "normal" for tri-iodothyronine, it is important to take age into account.

Adrenal Cortex

As noted above, the circadian variation in serum cortisol concentrations persists with ageing but there is a reduction in the 24-h excretion of urinary corticosteroid metabolites, suggesting that there may be a reduction in cortisol synthesis in the elderly. Ageing also is associated with a decline in the metabolic clearance of cortisol (Everitt 1980). Under conditions of stress, however, there is no evidence of a diminished adrenocortical reserve and indeed a standard dose of ACTH often produces a higher peak plasma concentration of cortisol in old age than in youth.

After the menopause a decline in ovarian function results in the adrenal cortex becoming the principal source of oestrogens and androgens. Thereafter there is a continuing decline in the cortical synthesis of steroids such as dehydro-epiandrosterone, 17-hydroxypregnenolone and pregnenolone; whereas there is an actual increase in androstenedione, 17-hydroxyprogesterone and progesterone production.

Gonadal Function in Women

After the menopause there is a dramatic fall in both oestrone and oestradiol (Chakravarti et al. 1976) (Fig. 1.2). Thereafter there is a further progressive decline in oestrone levels whereas oestradiol levels remain unchanged or even rise marginally. The effects of these changes on physiological function in general and bone metabolism are discussed in Chaps. 6 and 7.

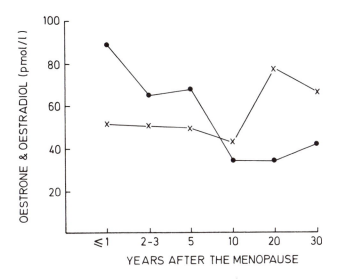

Fig. 1.2. Geometric mean concentrations of oestrone (*circles*) and oestradiol (*crosses*) in women after the menopause. The geometric mean concentrations of oestrone and oestradiol before the menopause are 439 pmol/l and 250 pmol/l. (After Chakravati et al. 1976.)

After the menopause there is a change in androgen levels, characterised by a decline in the serum androstenedione to 40% of the initial concentration (Studd and Thom 1981). In contrast, testosterone levels remain unaffected and its metabolism may contribute to the maintenance of 17-beta-oestradiol concentrations. The clinical relevance of these changes is uncertain.

Gonadal Function in Men

There is conflicting evidence on whether or not serum testosterone levels decline with increasing age and this may in part relate to whether populations studied have been healthy and living at home, or disabled and institutionalised (Vermeulen et al. 1972; Tsitouras et al. 1982). Recent work suggests, however, that both serum free and total testosterone concentrations are consistently reduced in the old. Conversely, there is no change in dihydrotestosterone concentrations (Desylpere and Vermeulen 1984).

The testis also secretes oestradiol, and plasma levels of this have been reported as being either normal or increased in old age (Pirke and Doerr 1973; Desylpere and Vermeulen 1984). This is associated with a consistent reduction in the ratio of testosterone to oestradiol, and is the result of either a reduction in oestradiol metabolism or an increase in the peripheral conversion of testosterone to oestradiol. Whatever the cause, the reduced testosterone to oestradiol ratio has been implicated as a potential cause of gynaecomastia in elderly men.

In a study of orchidectomy specimens it was found that in patients of up to 80 years of age with normal testicular histology and spermatogenesis, hormonal parameters were similar to those of younger men. In another group between the ages of 50 and 60 years, there was a significant fall in serum testosterone concentrations associated with a diminished testicular volume, reduced numbers of Sertoli, Leydig and germ cells, and increased plasma levels of LH and FSH. Thus there may be two populations of elderly males, one maintaining normal pituitary/gonadal axis function into advanced old age (Pamagna et al. 1987).

Calcium Homeostasis

Calcium balance is dependent upon a complex interaction between the parathyroid glands, the kidneys, the small bowel and bone. In essence, the parathyroid gland responds to hypocalcaemia by increasing parathyroid hormone (PTH) secretion. This in turn increases the renal conversion of 25-hydroxycholecalciferol (calcidiol) to 1,25-dihydroxycholecalciferol (calcitriol). The latter increases calcium absorption from the gut, increasing serum calcium levels and thus suppressing parathyroid gland activity. Secondary effects are that both PTH and calcitriol promote the resorption of skeletal calcium, and that PTH reduces the renal tubular resorption of phosphate.

Since ageing affects all four organ sites, it is often difficult to determine the primary site of age related changes in calcium metabolism. A number of investigations have shown a progressive rise in PTH levels with advancing age (Chapuy et al. 1983; Marcus et al. 1984; Orwoll and Muir 1986). PTH levels are also increased where age is associated with diminished renal function. The effect of PTH on the kidney, judged by urinary cyclic AMP concentrations, does not appear to diminish with ageing (Marcus et al. 1984; Orwoll and Muir 1986).

Studies on the effect of ageing on vitamin D and its metabolites vary, depending upon whether study groups were healthy and living at home, or infirm and institutionalised. There is a marginal reduction in 25-hydroxyvitamin D (calcidiol) levels in healthy old people, but most remain within normal limits (Orwoll and Muir 1986). Institutionalised individuals often have subnormal levels, and what little calcidiol remains is derived from diet rather than sunlight exposure.

Calcitriol levels are reduced in all categories of the elderly (Clemens et al. 1986; Dandona et al. 1986). There is uncertainty as to whether this is the result of reduced supplies of the precursor calcidiol, or whether it follows a reduction in the conversion of calcidiol to cacitriol by ageing kidneys.

Low serum calcitriol levels in old age result in a reduction in the gastro-intestinal absorption of calcium. A more important effect of the reduced calcium absorption is a decline in vertebral bone mineral content.

Fluid and Electrolyte Balance

Fluid Balance

A range of factors is responsible for the fact that old people are at increased risk of developing dehydration. The first is that they have an elevated thirst threshold (Phillips et al. 1984). Old men deprived of water for 24 h are less thirsty and drink less than younger counterparts.

The effect of ageing on posterior pituitary function is more complex. Thus, in old age, secretion of vasopressin (antidiuretic hormone) in response to a standard infusion of hypertonic saline is increased (Heldeman et al. 1978). Alcohol infusion, however, suppresses vasopressin secretion in all age groups, but only has a sustained effect in young people. In the elderly there is a paradoxical rise in vasopressin levels after the first half-hour of the infusion.

Vasopressin secretion is also influenced by changes in the blood pressure and circulating volume, but, while changing from a supine to an erect posture produces increased plasma vasopressin levels in young and elderly subjects, the effect is less pronounced in old age (Rowe et al. 1982). Nonetheless, elderly patients with dehydration are able to secrete sufficient vasopressin to achieve similar blood levels to those of young adults (Kirkland et al. 1984).

Fluid balance in the elderly is also critically affected by changes in renal function. The most important of these is that the capacity of renal distal tubules to conserve water is impaired (Rowe et al. 1976) (Table 1.2). The effect of exogen-

Table 1.2. Effect of water deprivation on urine osmolality (Rowe 1976)

Age (years)	Urine osmolality (mosmol/kg) Mean (SEM)	
	0–3 hours after deprivation	6–12 hours after deprivation
30–39	969 (41)	1109 (22)
40–59	949 (39)	1051 (19)
60–79	852 (64)	882 (49)

ous vasopressin on renal tubules is also diminished in old age (Lindeman et al. 1966). The practical consequence of these changes is that old people have a diminished fluid balance reserve, so that stroke patients with swallowing difficulties may rapidly become dehydrated or a relatively mild gastro-enteritis may cause severe dehydration.

Age changes in renal function noted from cross-sectional studies of subjects of different ages may give a false impression on the effects of ageing on the renal function of individuals. A longitudinal study showed that the creatinine clearance rate usually declined with increased age, but it remained unaltered in a third of subjects, and it actually increased in several (Lindeman et al. 1985). It should also be recognised that age changes are compounded by common disorders such as hypertension, diabetes and pyelonephritis.

Electrolyte Balance

Old people have an increased renal clearance of sodium, related mainly to reduced reabsorption of this from the distal tubule (Nunez et al. 1978). When placed on a low sodium diet, old people took twice as long to reduce their sodium excretion as young subjects (Epstein and Hollenberg 1976). This puts them at increased risk of developing hyponatraemia in sodium-depleting disorders such as gastro-enteritis.

Even in subjects with good health, there is a decline in intracellular potassium concentrations with increasing age (MacLennan 1986). This is probably related to a decline in physical activity rather than a reduced intake or a change in renal tubular function. Plasma potassium is unchanged or even increased in old age.

There is little information on the effects of ageing on magnesium status, but recently developed techniques for measuring electrolyte concentrations within lymphocytes may be of considerable value in this field.

Regulation of Blood Pressure

The humoral regulation of blood pressure is partly dependent upon a complex interaction between renin, angiotensin and aldosterone (Fig. 1.3). Plasma concentrations of these substances change in old age, but it is difficult to separate cause from effect, and the effects of ageing from those of disease.

There is evidence of a decline in plasma active renin levels with increasing age even in normotensive subjects (Crane and Harris 1976) (Fig. 1.4). Ageing has a similar effect on renin levels in patients with hypertension (Skott and Giesse 1983). However, analysis is hampered by the fact that there are problems of standardising the conditions under which renin assays are estimated, and that there has been a paucity of people over the age of 60 years included in studies. Possible reasons for the decline are reduced conversion of inactive renin, a decrease in the responsiveness of juxtaglomerular cells to sympathetic stimulation or increased fractional sodium delivery to the macula densa of the distal tubules.

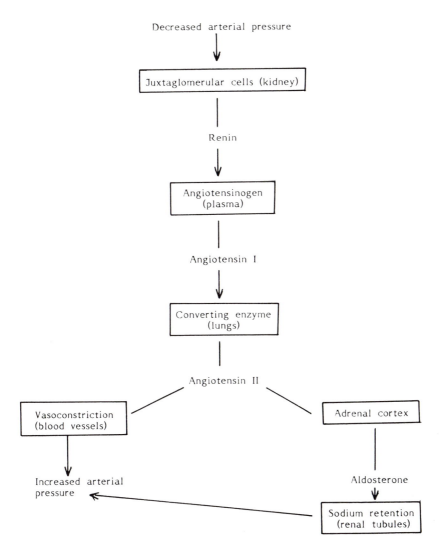

Fig. 1.3. Renin, angiotensin and aldosterone system.

There have been few studies of angiotensin levels in old age. One showed that, between the ages of 15 and 70, there was a progressive, but marginal rise in plasma renin substrate (angiotensinogen) levels (Immonon et al. 1981). However, neither the numbers of subjects nor their clinical status was defined so that the significance of the observations is doubtful.

In both men and women there is a decline in the 24-h urinary excretion of aldosterone with increasing age (Fig. 1.5) (Crane and Harris 1976). Plasma aldosterone concentrations tend to decline with age and correlate with plasma renin activity

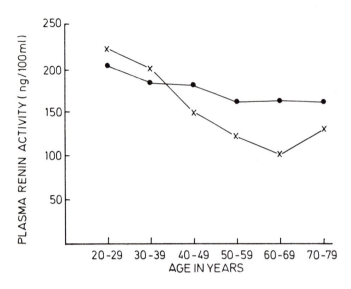

Fig. 1.4. Age and plasma renin activity in men (*circles*) and women (*crosses*). (After Crane and Harris 1976.)

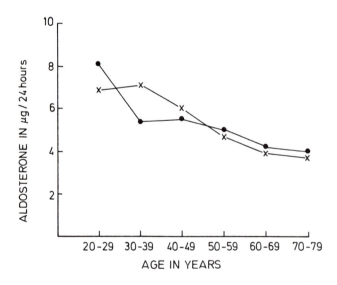

Fig. 1.5. Age and 24-h urinary excretion of aldosterone in men (*circles*) and women (*crosses*). (After Crane and Harris 1976.)

(Tsunoda et al. 1986). It is not clear whether the reduction of aldosterone secretion is a secondary effect of reduced renin and angiotensin activity, or whether it also represents a change in the sensitivity of the adrenal cortex to angiotensin II.

Adrenal medullary function is unimpaired in the elderly as judged by plasma adrenaline concentrations and adrenaline secretion rates (Morrow et al. 1987). Peak plasma noradrenaline levels in response to an upright posture or oral glucose are substantially higher in healthy people over 65 than in their younger counterparts (Young et al. 1980). Plasma noradrenaline but not adrenaline clearance is significantly reduced in elderly subjects compared with young ones (Morrow et al. 1987).

The question arises as to whether the various changes in renin, aldosterone and catecholamine activity in the elderly bear any relationship to the high prevalence of both hypertension and postural hypotension in this group. An investigation of elderly patients with hypertension revealed that although their plasma renin concentrations were reduced (low-renin hypertension) they had a disproportionately low renal blood flow and elevated peripheral and renal vascular resistance (Messerli et al. 1983). In these circumstances it seems likely that low plasma renin levels are the result of impaired juxtaglomerular function, and that the high peripheral resistance is due to an elevation of plasma catecholamines.

Whereas in most young patients orthostatic hypotension is the result of autonomic degeneration, there is no evidence that such is the case in the elderly. Indeed, the plasma catecholamine response to changes in posture is similar in elderly patients with orthostatic hypotension to that in controls (Robinson et al. 1983). Here again it seems likely that reduced arterial compliance is the main culprit.

Carbohydrate Metabolism

There is overwhelming evidence that with increasing age there is a decline in glucose utilisation associated with impairment of glucose tolerance (Davidson, 1979; Jackson et al. 1982). Old age, however, is compounded by a high prevalence of chronic disease, obesity and drug treatment.

In one comparison between young controls and healthy, ambulant and non-obese elderly subjects, means and standard errors of fasting blood glucose for the two groups were 4.7 ± 0.1 and 5.2 ± 0.1 mmol/l respectively (Rosenthal et al. 1982). Sixty minutes after the oral administration of 75 g of glucose the difference in blood glucose levels between the two groups was only 1 mmol/l. Thus, the effects of ageing on carbohydrate metabolism are minimal compared with those of disease and drug therapy.

Ageing has little effect on the secretion of insulin by islet cells. Fasting plasma insulin levels are not reduced and, indeed, may be marginally increased in old age (Reaven and Reaven 1985). Ageing is also associated with an increased insulin response to an oral glucose load (Chlouverakis et al. 1967). The effects of age on the secretion of insulin in response to a continuous intravenous infusion of glucose have also been investigated (Ratzmann et al. 1982). Here, both the initial and delayed insulin responses to glucose infusion are marginally reduced, but not sufficiently to account for differences in glucose metabolism in the elderly. In aged rats the capacity of individual islet cells to secrete insulin is impaired, but there is a cellular hyperplasia which compensates for this (Reaven and Reaven 1985). As yet, there have been no studies to confirm that these age changes occur in humans. Ageing has no effect on the metabolic clearance rate of insulin (Ratzmann et al. 1982).

There have been conflicting results on the effects of ageing on glucagon secretion. In one study of subjects between the ages of 20 and 69, there was a rise in plasma glucagon levels with increasing age (Berger et al. 1978). Multiple regression analysis suggested that the increased glucagon levels were the result of an increase in percentage body fat in old age, so that it was obesity rather than age which was responsible for the effect (Elahi et al. 1982). The reason for a relationship between high plasma glucagon levels and obesity has not yet been elucidated.

Most studies have found no relationship between age and plasma growth hormone levels (Berger et al. 1978). In one, in which there was an apparent inverse relationship, the effect was probably the result of an inverse association between low growth hormone levels and an increase in total body fat in old age (Rudman et al. 1981).

In summary then, there is little evidence that impaired glucose tolerance is the result of changes in islet cell or anterior pituitary function in old age. This raises the question as to whether there is a change in the responsiveness of tissues to hormones. This can be tested by measuring the rate at which glucose has to be infused intravenously to maintain the blood glucose at a steady level of hyperglycaemia (hyperglycaemic clamp) and relating this to plasma insulin levels. An alternative is to infuse insulin to maintain a steady elevated plasma insulin level, and to then measure the amount of glucose which has to be given intravenously to maintain baseline blood glucose levels (euglycaemic clamp). Again, the ratio of glucose infused to insulin levels is calculated. In both instances the ratio of glucose metabolised per unit of insulin is substantially lower in elderly subjects (De Fronzo 1979). This relative insulin resistance is also demonstrated by a reduced rate of fall of plasma glucose in response to insulin infusion (Ratzmann et al. 1982).

A variety of factors have been adduced as causes for the change in tissue sensitivity to insulin (Davidson 1979). One is that there might be a reduced carbohydrate intake by old people so that their tissues become less efficient at metabolising glucose. Another is that old people have a lower level of physical activity so that they utilise less glucose. In addition, they have a reduced lean body mass so that less muscle is available for glucose uptake. At the tissue level, it has been shown that the peripheral glucose uptake by forearm muscle is diminished in healthy elderly individuals (Jackson et al. 1982). Abnormalities in the insulin molecule synthesised, an increase in circulating insulin antagonists, and defects in insulin activity at receptor or post-receptor sites have also been proposed.

Support for the first of the last three possibilities is that, in the elderly, an increased proportion of circulating insulin is in the form of pro-insulin, the less active precursor of insulin (Duckworth et al. 1972) although C peptide to insulin ratios are unchanged (Jackson et al. 1982). There is no evidence that insulin antagonism by counterregulatory hormones is a problem in old age. Finally, in fat cells at least, there is a substantial reduction in the number of insulin receptor sites in samples taken from elderly subjects (Giafranco et al. 1981). There is thus a receptor defect and there is also evidence for a post-receptor defect in the insulin response from fat cells from obese elderly subjects (Lonnroth and Smith 1986).

It is believed that a complex of chromium and nicotinic acid is in some way involved in the facilitation of insulin binding to receptors and it has recently been observed in elderly humans that dietary supplementation with chromium and nicotinic acid improved glucose tolerance (Urberg et al. 1987).

Lipid Metabolism

Ageing is associated with an increase in the proportion of the body composed of fat. This is partly due to a decline in lean body mass, but in many people there is also an increase in fat deposition (Heber and Bray 1980). These changes occur despite the fact that, with increasing age, there is a progressive decline in calorie intake (Committee on Medical Aspects of Food Policy 1979). A more likely explanation is that, in most individuals, there is a decline in energy expenditure from early adult life onwards (Shepard 1978). Even at rest there is a decline in the basal metabolic rate of old people (Tzankoff and Norris 1978).

The decline in metabolic rate is partly related to the reduction in lean body mass associated with ageing, but changes in nutrient metabolism may also be important. An example is that, in old age, the calorie expenditure following a standard dose of oral glucose is reduced (Golaz et al. 1983). Possible factors involved in this change include a reduced lipogenic enzyme response to glucose, and a less striking sympathetic autonomic response to meals in old age (Kaiser et al. 1983). Cross-sectional studies have also demonstrated a rise in both serum cholesterol and triglyceride concentrations with increasing age (Bierman 1984). These changes are probably related to an increase in the incidence of obesity, since in this condition there is an increase in the synthesis of both cholesterol and triglyceride. Despite the increased prevalence of both hyperlipidaemia and atherosclerosis in old age, the importance of hyperlipidaemia as a risk factor in conditions such as coronary artery disease declines with age.

Thymus

The thymus, in addition to processing lymphocytes, secretes a variety of polypeptide hormones including thymopoietin. The latter has an important role in the differentiation of precursors into mature lymphocytes (Weksler 1983). Since there is involution of the thymus with age, it is not surprising that there is a parallel decline in plasma levels of thymopoietin (Lewis et al. 1978). It is tempting to attribute the signs of immunological incompetence, often found in old people, to thymopoietin deficiency. However, other explanations, such as exhaustion of T-cell precursors in the bone marrow, are more likely.

References

Arnetz BB, Lahnberg G, Eneroth P, Thunell S (1984) Age-related differences in the serum prolactin responses during standardised surgery. Life Sci 35: 2675–2680

Berger D, Crowther RC, Floyd JC et al. (1978) Effect of ageing on fasting plasma levels of pancreatic hormones in man. J Clin Endocrinol Metab 47: 1183–1189

Bierman EL (1984) Ageing and atherosclerosis In: Stout RW (ed) Arterial disease in the elderly. Churchill Livingstone, Edinburgh, pp 17–31

Caplan RH, Wickus G, Glasser JE et al. (1981) Serum concentrations of the iodothyronines in elderly subjects: decreased triiodothyronine (T_3) and free T_3 index. J Am Geriatr Soc 29: 19–24

Chakravarti S, Collins WP, Forecast JD et al. (1976) Hormonal profiles after the menopause. Br Med J 2: 784–786

Chapuy M, Durr F, Chapuy P (1983) Age-related changes in parathyroid hormone and 25 hydroxy-cholecalciferol levels. J Gerontol 38: 19–22

Chlouverakis C, Jarrett RJ, Keen H (1967) Glucose tolerance, age, and circulating insulin. Lancet I: 806–809

Clemens TL, Zhou XY, Myler M et al. (1986) Serum vitamin D_2 and vitamin D_3 metabolite concentrations and absorption of vitamin D_2 in elderly subjects. J Clin Endocrinol Metab 63: 656–660

Committee on Medical Aspects of Food Policy (1979) Nutrition and health in old age. HMSO, London

Crane MG, Harris JJ (1976) Effect of ageing on renin activity and aldosterone excretion. J Lab Clin Med 87: 946–959

Dandona P, Menon K, Shenoz R et al. (1986) Low 1,25-dihydroxyvitamin D secondary hyper-parathyroidism, and normal osteocalcin in elderly subjects. J Clin Endocrinol Metab 63: 459–462

Davidson MB (1979) The effect of ageing on carbohydrate metabolism: A review of the English literature and a practical approach to the diagnosis of diabetes mellitus in the elderly. Metabolism 28: 688–705

De Fronzo RA (1979) Glucose intolerance and ageing. Diabetes 28: 1096–1101

Deslypere JP, Vermeulen A (1984) Leydig cell function in normal men: effect of age: life style, residence, diet and activity. J Clin Endocrinol Metab 59: 955–962

Dilman V (1976) The hypothalamic control of ageing and age-associated pathology. The elevation mechanism of ageing. In: Everitt AV, Burgess JA, Thomas J (eds) Hypothalamus, pituitary and ageing. Springfield, pp 634–667

Duckworth WC, Kitabchi AE, Heinemann M (1972) Direct measurement of plasma proinsulin in normal and diabetic subjects. Am J Med 53: 418–426

Elahi D, Muller DC, Tzankoff SP et al. (1982) Effect of age and obesity on fasting levels of glucose, insulin, glucagon, and growth hormone in man. J Gerontol 37: 385–391

Epstein M, Hollenberg NK (1976) Age as a determinant of renal sodium conservation in normal men. J Lab Clin Med 87: 411–417

Everitt AV (1980) The neuroendocrine system and ageing. Gerontology 26: 108–119

Florini JR, Prinz PN, Vitiello MV, Hintz RL (1985) Sonatamedin levels in healthy young and old men – relationship to peak and 24 hour integrated levels of growth hormone. J Gerontol 40: 2–7

Giafranco P, Cassader M, Diana A et al. (1981) Insulin resistance in the aged: the role of the peripheral insulin receptors. Metabolism 30: 46–49

Golaz A, Schutz Y, Broqhet C et al. (1983) Decreased thermogenic response to an oral glucose load in older subjects. J Am Geriatr Soc 31: 144–148

Govoni S, Pasinetti G, Trabucchi M et al. (1983) Plasma prolactin concentrations in a large population of healthy old people. Br Med J 287: 1107

Harman SM, Wehmann RE, Blackman MR (1984) Pituitary thyroid hormone economy in healthy ageing men: basal indices of thyroid function and thyrotrophin responses to constant infusion of thyrotrophin releasing hormone. J Clin Endocrinol Metab 58: 320–326

Heber D, Bray GA (1980) Energy requirements In: Exton-Smith AN, Caird FI (eds) Metabolic and nutritional disorders in the elderly. John Wright, Bristol, pp 1–12

Heldeman JH, Vestal RE, Rowe JW et al. (1978) The response of arginine vasopressin to intravenous ethanol and hypertonic saline in man: the impact of ageing. J Gerontol 33: 39–47

Immonon I, Fyhrquist F, Pohjavuori M, Simell O (1981) Age dependence of human plasma renin substrate. Scand J Clin Lab Invest 41: 167–170

Imura M (1985) ACTH and related peptides. Clin Endocrinol Metab 14: 845–856

Jackson RA, Blix PM, Mathews JA et al. (1982) Influence of ageing on glucose homeostasis. J Clin Endocrinol Metab 55: 840–848

Kaiser FE, Schwartz HL, Mariash CN, Oppenheimer JH (1983) Comparison of age-related decreases in the basal and carbohydrate inducible levels of lipogenic enzymes in adipose tissue and liver. Metabolism 32: 838–845

Kaler LW, Gliesman P, Craven J et al. (1986) Loss of enhanced nocturnal growth hormone secretion in ageing rhesus males. Endocrinology 119: 1281–1284

Kirkland J, Lye M, Goddard C et al. (1984) Plasma arginine vasopressin in dehydrated elderly patients. Clin Endocrinol Metab 20: 451–456

Lang I, Schernthaner G, Pietschmann P et al. (1987) Effects of sex and age on growth hormone response to growth hormone releasing hormone in healthy individuals. J Clin Endocrinol Metab 65: 535–540

Lewis VM, Twomey JJ, Bealmear P et al. (1978) Age, thymic involution and circulating thymic hormone activity. J Clin Endocrinol Metab 47: 145–150

Lindeman RD, Lee TD, Yiengst MY, Shock NW (1966) Influence of age, renal disease, hypertension, diuretics and calcium on the anti-diuretic responses to suboptimal infusion of vasopressin. J Clin Lab Med 68: 206–223

Lindeman RD, Tobin J, Shock NW (1985) Longitudinal studies on the rate of decline in renal function with age. J Am Geriatr Soc 33: 278–285

Lonnroth P, Smith V (1986) Ageing enhances the insulin resistance in obesity through both receptor and post receptor alterations. J Clin Endocrinol Metab 62: 433–437

Lye M (1984) Electrolyte disorders in the elderly. Clin Endocrinol Metab 13: 377–398

MacLennan WJ (1986) Diuretic therapy and potassium balance. In: Swift CG (ed) Clinical pharmacology in the elderly. Marcel Dekker, New York, pp 179–211

Marcus R, Madvig P, Young G (1984) Age-related changes in parathyroid hormone and parathyroid hormone action in normal humans. J Clin Endocrinol Metab 58: 223–230

Messerli FZ, Ventura HO, Glade LB et al. (1983) Essential hypertension in the elderly: haemodynamics, intravascular volume, plasma renin activity, and circulating catecholamine levels. Lancet II: 983–985

Mills TM, Mahesh VB (1977) Gonadotrophin secretion in the menopause. Obstet Gynecol 4: 71–84

Morrow LA, Linares OA, Hill TK et al. (1987) Age differences in the plasma clearance mechanisms for epinephrine and norepinephrine in humans. J Clin Endocrinol Metab 65: 508–511

Muta K, Kato K, Akamine Y, Ibayashi H (1981) Age-related changes in the feedback regulation of gonadotrophin secretion by sex steroids in men. Acta Endocrinol (Copenh) 96: 154–162

Nunez JFM, Iglesias CG, Roman AB et al. (1978) Renal handling of sodium in old people: a functional study. Age Ageing 7: 178–181

Ordene KW, Pan C, Barzel US, Surks MI (1983) Variable thyrotrophin response to thyrotrophin releasing hormone after small decreases in plasma thyroid hormone concentrations in patients with advanced age. Metabolism 32: 881–888

Orwoll ES, Muir DE (1986) Alterations in calcium, vitamin D, and parathyroid hormone physiology in normal men with ageing: relationship to the development of senile osteopenia. J Clin Endocrinol Metab 63: 1262–1269

Parker CR, Porter JC (1984) Luteinising hormone releasing hormone and thyrotrophin releasing hormone in the hypothalamus of women – effects of age and reproductive status. J Clin Endocrinol Metab 58: 488–491

Pamagna R, Martin A, Nistal M, Amal P (1987) Testicular involution in elderly men: comparison of histologic qualitative studies with human performance. Fertil Steril 47: 671–679

Pavlov EP, Harman SM, Merriam GR, Gelato MC, Blackman MR (1986) Responses of growth hormone and somatomedin-C to GH-releasing hormone in healthy ageing men. J Clin Endocrinol Metab 62: 595–600

Phillips PA, Rolls BJ, Ledingham JGG et al. (1984) Reduced thirst after water deprivation in healthy elderly men. New Engl J Med 311: 753–759

Pirke KM, Doerr P (1973) Age related changes and interrelationships between plasma testosterone, oestradiol, and testosterone binding globulin in normal adult males. Acta Endocrinol (Copenh) 74: 792–800

Prinz PN, Weitzman ED, Cunningham GR, Karacan I (1983) Plasma growth hormone during sleep in young and aged men. J Gerontol 38: 519–524

Ratzmann KP, Witt S, Heinke P, Schulz B (1982) The effect of ageing on insulin sensitivity and insulin secretion in non-obese healthy subjects. Acta Endocrinol (Copenh) 100: 543–549

Reaven GM, Reaven EP (1985) Age, glucose intolerance, and non-insulin-dependent diabetes mellitus. J Am Geriatr Soc 33: 286–290

Robinson BJ, Johnson RH, Lambie DG, Palmer KT (1983) Do elderly patients with an excessive fall of blood pressure on standing have evidence of autonomic failure? Clin Sci 64: 587–591

Rolandi E, Franceschini R, Marabini A et al. (1987) Twenty-four hour beta-endorphin secretory pattern in the elderly. Acta Endocrinol (Copenh) 115: 441–446

Rosenthal M, Doheme L, Greenfield M et al. (1982) Effect of age on glucose tolerance, insulin secretion, and in vivo insulin action. J Am Geriatr Soc 30: 562–567

Rowe JW, Shock NW, de Fronzo RA (1976) The influence of age on the renal response to water deprivation in man. Nephron 17: 270–278

Rowe JW, Minaker KL, Sparrow D, Robertson GL (1982) Age-related failure of volume-pressure-mediated vasopressin release. J Clin Endocrinol Metab 54: 661–664

Rudman D, Kutner MH, Rogers CM et al. (1981) Impaired growth hormone secretion in the adult population: relation to age and adiposity. J Clin Invest 67: 1361–1369

Sawin CT, Chopra D, Azizi F et al. (1979) The ageing thyroid. JAMA 242: 247–250

Shepard RJ (1978) Physical activity and ageing. Croom Helm, London, pp 146–175

Shibasaki T, Shizume K, Nakahara M et al. (1984) Age-related changes in plasma growth hormone; response to growth hormone-releasing factor in man. J Clin Endocrinol Metab 58: 212–214

Skott P, Giese J (1983) Age and the renin-angiotensin system. Acta Med Scand (Suppl) 676: 45–49

Studd JW, Thom MH (1981) Ovarian failure and ageing. Clin Endocrinol Metab 10: 89–113

Tointon Y, Fevre M, Bogdan A et al. (1984) Patterns of plasma melatonin with ageing: Stability of nychtohemoral rhythms and differences in seasonal variations. Acta Endocrinol (Copenh) 106: 145–151

Tsitouras PD, Martin CE, Harman SM (1982) Relationship of serum testosterone to sexual activity in healthy elderly men. J Gerontol 37: 288–293

Tsunoda K, Abe K, Goto T et al. (1986) Effect of age on the renin angiotensin aldosterone system, in normal subjects. Simultaneous measurement of active and inactive renin substrate and aldosterone in plasma. J Clin Endocrinol Metab 62: 384–389

Tzankoff SP, Norris AH (1978) Longitudinal changes in basal metabolism in man. J Appl Physiol 45: 536–539

Urberg M, Zemel MB (1987) Evidence for synergism between chromium and nicotinic acid in the control of glucose tolerance in elderly humans. Metabolism 36: 896–899

Vermeulen A, Rubens R, Verdonck L (1972) Testosterone secretion and metabolism in male senescence. J Clin Endocrinol Metab 34: 730–735

Weizmann A, Weizmann R, Hart S et al. (1983) The correlation of increased serum prolactin levels with decreased sexual desire and activity in elderly men. J Am Geriatr Soc 31: 485–488

Weksler ME (1983) The thymus gland and ageing. Ann Intern Med 98: 105–107

Young JB, Rowe JW, Pallotta JA et al. (1980) Enhanced plasma norepinephine response to upright posture and oral glucose administration in elderly human subjects. Metabolism 29: 532–539

2 The Clinical Assessment of Endocrine Disorders in the Elderly

The signs and symptoms of endocrine disorders are often subtle and insidious in onset, so a careful history and physical examination is particularly important. The many biochemical tests now available should be used with economy and acumen. Clinicians dealing with old people have the additional problems that the history may be long and rambling, that deafness, dysarthria or dysphasia may block communication, and that weariness in the patient, or even the examiner, may intervene. These difficulties are compounded in the minority of old people with mental impairment.

A problem of more particular relevance to endocrine disorders is the considerable overlap between the clinical features of endocrine disorders, and those of ageing itself. Again a wide range of factors including an increased visceral pain threshold, impaired immunological function, or even a stoical attitude to ill health result in symptoms of endocrine disease often being absent, vague or atypical in old people.

History

Ageing is traditionally associated with apathy and a deterioration in mobility. In reality these are invariably the result of mental or physical ill health so that careful clinical assessment is indicated. A metabolic or endocrine disorder often presents in this way, but since apathetic patients rarely complain, and deterioration is insidious, it may go undiagnosed for years, until an intervening social or medical crisis exacerbates the picture.

Only a minority of old people with hypothyroidism have the clinical features of myxoedema, so that any elderly woman with an unexplained deterioration in vitality should have blood taken for assessment of thyroid function. The clinical manifestations of non-insulin dependent diabetes may also be vague. Indeed, they are often only recognised in retrospect, when correction of an elevated blood glucose concentration produces an improvement in alertness and agility. The role of electrolyte depletion is more controversial. Some clinicians produced evidence that dietary deficiency of potassium was an important cause of mental and physical incapacity, but their findings have not been confirmed, and it now seems likely that potassium depletion is only important in patients on diuretics with severe hypokalaemia (MacLennan 1981). Hyponatraemia and hypomagnesaemia may also cause lethargy, but their importance in old age has not been evaluated yet.

Endocrine disease in the elderly may produce any of the symptoms occurring in younger patients, but these are frequently absent. An example is that hyperthyroidism is less likely to present with anxiety, tremor, excessive sweating, and diarrhoea (Davis and Davis 1974). Again the advent of multichannel analysers has increased the frequency of diagnosis of hypercalcaemia in elderly patients. However, few of these develop the classical mental disorders, gastro-intestinal disturbance, or bone pain (Paterson and MacLennan 1984).

Diagnosis is further confounded by the problem of multiple pathology. Thus hypothyroidism may cause constipation, but the association may be masked by the effects of anticholinergic drugs, reduced mobility and dehydration. Again hypothyroid patients often have a preference for a heated environment, but old people in general are notoriously bad at regulating the temperature of their environment. This characteristically puts them at risk from hypothermia, but some go to the opposite extreme and live in a hothouse environment.

Mental Function

Mental Impairment

People of increasing age show only minor changes in mental function, and many of these are probably the result of differences in generation cohorts rather than ageing. Conversely, mental illness is common in old age and is a major cause of psychological and social incapacity.

Acute confusional states are due to acute physical illness or drug toxicity. The two most common causes of chronic mental impairment are Alzheimer's disease or multiple cerebral infarcts, with a small but important minority being due to more reversible physical disorders (Tomlinson et al. 1970) (Table 2.1). In addition, mental incapacity is often accentuated by chronic physical illnesses, or inappropriate medication. Endocrine disorders or hormonal treatment should always be considered as culprits, since, once identified, they are often easily treated.

Most hypothyroid patients have some degree of mental impairment, but in old age, the clinical picture is complicated by the high prevalence of other disorders interfering with cerebral activity. Examples include Parkinsonism, cerebrovascu-

Table 2.1. Pathological basis of dementia (Tomlinson et al. 1970)

Alzheimer's disease	50%
Alzheimer's disease and multiple cerebral infarcts	20%
Multiple cerebral infarcts	20%
Other lesions	10%

Table 2.2. Characteristics of apathetic thyrotoxicosis (Thomas et al. 1970)

Clinical features	Classical thyrotoxicosis	Apathetic thyrotoxicosis
Age (years)	36.0 (15.8)	67.7 (13.9)
Duration of symptoms (months)	8.0 (3.9)	25.6 (32.6)
Weight change (kg)	−4.9 (6.4)	−17.3 (4.7)

lar disease and nutritional deficiency. This means that treatment with thyroxine does not always reverse the dementia. Occasionally a patient may present with the classical picture of myxoedema madness in which there are depression, agitation, paranoia, delusions and hallucinations. This usually responds well to replacement therapy.

Many old people with hyperthyroidism, far from being hyperactive and agitated, are withdrawn and apathetic. The condition has been labelled as apathetic thyrotoxicosis (Thomas et al. 1970) (Table 2.2). Often the only other systemic effect is profound weight loss. In fact the picture is frequently mistaken for the extreme state of neglect often associated with severe senile or multi-infarct dementia.

Corticosteroid excess often produces bizarre changes in the mental function of old people (Ling et al. 1981). These include paranoid delusions, hallucinations, disorientation and agitated confusion. The diagnosis should be obvious if symptoms follow the administration of large doses of corticosteroids. It is more easily missed if, due to the inappropriate secretion of ACTH from a tumour, the condition develops so rapidly that the more florid physical signs of Cushing's syndrome have not had time to develop, and behavioural problems are wrongly attributed to cerebral metastases.

Diabetes mellitus may predispose to multiple cerebral infarctions associated with accelerated atherosclerosis (Wilkinson 1981). Again, sulphonylurea drugs, particularly the longer acting ones, may induce recurrent attacks of hypoglycaemia with confusion and impaired consciousness. More severe hypoglycaemia from the longer-acting sulphonylureas or from insulin may go on to produce focal areas of cortical necrosis, particularly at the bases of the sulci, so that mental impairment can be permanent.

Pancreatic islet cell tumours (insulinomas) are no more common in old age, but should be considered as an occasional cause of behavioural problems, and provide justification for checking blood glucose levels in elderly patients with mental impairment. One of the reasons for hypoglycaemia being missed in the elderly is that florid signs such as pallor, sweating and tachycardia are often masked by autonomic dysfunction associated with ageing, disease and polypharmacy.

Hyperparathyroidism causes mental confusion which can be reversed by reducing the serum calcium concentration (Paterson and MacLennan 1984). However, since dementia and hypercalcaemia are both common in old age they often occur coincidentally. Hypercalcaemia is unlikely to be the cause of mental impairment unless the serum calcium is in excess of 3.0 mmol/l. Hypocalcaemia may also interfere with mental function, and should always be considered in patients with a previous history of thyroidectomy who present with neuropsychiatric symptoms.

Depression

Ill health, social deprivation and age-related biochemical changes combine to pro-duce a high prevalence of depression in old age. In a minority, however, endocrine disorders are the root cause. Examples include hypoglycaemia and hyper-parathyroidism. Again, apathy associated with myxoedema or hyperthyroidism is often mistaken for depression. Finally, while corticosteroid therapy is useful in inducing mild euphoria, it can have the reverse effect.

There has been considerable interest in the role of corticosteroid intolerance, and the dexamethasone suppression test has been advocated as a biochemical index of depression (Carroll et al. 1981). However, there is too much overlap between depressed patients and controls for this to be of practical clinical value (American College of Physicians 1984).

Central Nervous System

Impairment of Conscious Level and Coma

The effects of ageing and multiple diagnosis can mask the clinical features of endocrine disorders, so that they may present for the first time as a coma. An example is myxoedema coma, a relatively rare condition which usually occurs in the elderly (Forester 1963). Apart from being comatose or lethargic, patients have a low central body temperature, dry pale skin, and sluggish tendon reflexes. The main differential diagnosis is that of hypothermia due to other causes, and there is considerable overlap between the signs of hypothermia and ageing and those of myxoedema. The only distinguishing feature is that in hypothermia the contrac-tion and relaxation phases of the ankle reflex are delayed, whereas in myxoedema only the relaxation phase is affected (MacLennan 1985). These can be accurately quantified using a photo-electric reflexometer. Unfortunately, many old people do not have an ankle reflex and in them the test is impracticable.

Coma may also be the result of uncontrolled diabetes mellitus. The classical presentation is that of diabetic ketoacidosis in which there is rapid deterioration often associated with vomiting, thirst, polydipsia, polyuria, abdominal discom-fort, rapid respiration and a smell of acetone on the breath. In old people, how-ever, deterioration is often insidious with a rise in blood glucose concentration, but little change in acid–base balance (hyperglycaemic hyperosmolar non-ketotic coma). Deterioration occurs over several days with gradual impairment of mental function and consciousness. Though the patient becomes severly dehydrated, it may be difficult to identify this in old age for reasons already discussed. Hypo-glycaemic coma may also be misdiagnosed because autonomic dysfunction in old age masks the more florid signs of this.

Past History

Even if an elderly patient is alert, he may have a long and convoluted past history, so that he may easily miss an essential piece of information, or the time sequence of the information may be incorrect. Old general practice or hospital records are a useful adjunct, but these are often overloaded, disorganised or microfilmed so that at a busy clinic there is the temptation not to delve too deeply and concentrate on more recent medical correspondence. Thus, impatience, rather than lack of clinical acumen, may lead to misdiagnosis.

A past history is particularly important in thyroid disease where a patient previously treated for hyperthyroidism, particularly with radio-iodine, may present many years later with hypothyroidism. Again, thyroidectomy may have caused damage to the parathyroid glands and be the explanation for hypocalcaemia. Finally, some elderly women with a goitre give a history of receiving iodine for the treatment of thyroid enlargement in adolescence.

Family History

As in any age group, there may be a family history of thyroid disease, hyperparathyroidism, pernicious anaemia or particularly diabetes mellitus, and this information can be useful for arriving at a diagnosis.

Dietary History

When obese elderly ladies are interrogated about their diet, they often deny excessive intake, and indeed sometimes suggest that they take less than non-obese contemporaries. There is the suspicion that they are often being dishonest, or that they have forgotten snacks taken between meals. Studies of elderly hospital inpatients, however, have established that there is little relation between calorie intake and body build (Fig. 2.1) (MacLennan et al. 1975). It is difficult to account for this finding. Most obese people have a higher basal metabolic rate than their

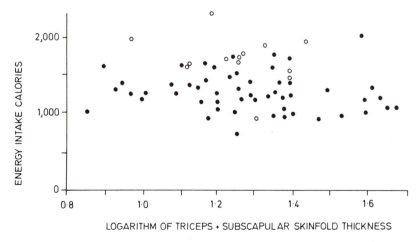

Fig. 2.1. Energy intake related to skinfold thickness. (After MacLennan et al. 1975.)

lean counterparts. It may be that obese elderly hospital patients, by virtue of disability, expend less energy in exercise. However, this has not been formally investigated.

Conversely, a low energy intake is a relatively uncommon cause of weight loss in old age. More important factors are increased catabolism associated with chronic sepsis or malignancy, or increased basal energy expenditure as in hyperthyroidism or Parkinson's disease.

Drug History

Hormonal imbalance is often the result of drug treatment in the elderly. A common example in elderly men is gynaecomastia. The explanation is obvious where a patient is receiving stilboestrol for carcinoma of the prostate, but a disparate range of other drugs many with antiandrogenic activity has been implicated (Table 2.3) (see Chap. 11).

Table 2.3. Drugs causing gynaecomastia

Oestrogens
Androgens
Spironolactone
Methyldopa
Cimetidine
Cardiac glycosides
Tricyclic antidepressants
Benzodiazepines
Phenothiazines
Isoniazid
Amphetamines
Cytotoxic agents

Drugs also may interfere with carbohydrate tolerance. Thus, corticosteroids have a direct effect on gluconeogenesis. In the case of thiazide diuretics, it has been argued that increased blood glucose concentrations are a consequence of potassium depletion (Heldeman et al. 1983). However, correction of the depletion has no effect on carbohydrate intolerance.

Drug therapy should be investigated in patients with a history of recent weight gain. Both phenothiazines and tricyclic antidepressants cause this by stimulating appetite and reducing physical activity, while corticosteroids have a direct effect on carbohydrate and fat metabolism.

Medication occasionally interferes with thyroid function. Amiodarone by virtue of the high iodine content of its molecule may produce either hypothyroidism or hyperthyroidism in up to 6% of patients (Wenzel 1981) (Chap. 3). Again, by increasing the metabolism of thyroxine and tri-iodothyronine, an anticonvulsant drug has occasionally been implicated as a cause of hypothyroidism. There is laboratory evidence that sulphonylureas have a goitrogenic effect, but in clinical practice hypothyroidism is no more common in patients on sulphonylureas than controls. Finally, a wide range of drugs, though modifying thyroid function tests, do not cause overt thyroid disease.

Physical Examination

Identification of the subtle signs of endocrine disease in old age requires detailed knowledge and experience of the effects of ageing on general appearance and organ function.

General Examination

The facial appearance of ageing is mainly the result of changes in the structure and physical properties of connective tissue. Prolonged exposure to sunlight accelerates the process, while treatment with oestrogens delays it. Local circulatory changes also may result in facial pallor, even where the haemoglobin concentration is satisfactory. These features of ageing are further accentuated, if because of apathy, depression or neurological disease the patient has little expression. There is considerable overlap between these changes and the sallow, puffy and expressionless face of hypothyroidism. Pallor of the skin may suggest hypopituitarism. Again, the craggy features of old men merge with the large nose, jaw and tongue associated with acromegaly.

The effects of ageing on hair should be distinguished from those of male pattern baldness which often occurs relatively early in life and has strong genetic associations. In old age hair is finer, more friable and more sparse. Hypothyroidism produces similar changes in which one of the few distinguishing features is a selective loss of hair from the outer third of the eyebrows. Another occasional cause of diffuse hair loss is ascorbic acid deficiency, one of the few situations in which a doctor can produce a guaranteed cure for baldness.

Hair depigmentation occurs at such a varible rate that it is of no value in establishing chronological age. However, endocrine disorders sometimes delay depigmentation. An example is that a high proportion of elderly hypothyroid patients have dark rather than grey hair (W. B. Wright, personal observation). Conversely, facial hirsutism in elderly women is a variant of normal, and is rarely associated with endocrine disease.

Ageing produces a wide range of changes in the eye, the most important of which are a loss of lens elasticity and increased lens opacity. In diabetes, opacification is accelerated so that cataracts may be encountered 10–20 years earlier than in other old people.

A further change in old age is that the pupil is smaller and reacts more sluggishly to light, probably a reflection of impaired autonomic function. This, combined with lens opacities, makes it extremely difficult to view the fundus in old people so that important changes such as those of diabetic retinopathy are easily missed. The problem is resolved by dilating the pupil with a short-acting mydriatic agent such as tropicamide. There is the theoretical risk of causing acute closed angle glaucoma, but, since in old age the more common form of the condition is chronic simple open angle glaucoma, mydriasis rarely causes problems.

Many old people exhibit a striking arcus senilis. Under the age of 40 this often indicates a severe hyperlipidaemia. In old age, however, the condition is associated with neither hyperlipidaemia nor atherosclerosis and is of no diagnostic or prognostic significance. This should be distinguished from the band keratopathy sometimes found in hyperparathyroidism in which opaque material is deposited near the limbus beneath Bowman's membrane.

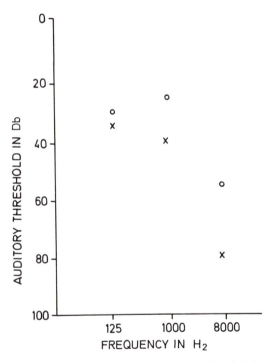

Fig. 2.2. Effect of ageing on auditory threshold for the left ear in women aged 65–74 (*open circles*) and 75 and over (*crosses*). (Personal data.)

Ageing is accompanied by an increased incidence of high tone deafness (Fig. 2.2). In hypothyroidism, cochlear, vestibular and neuronal damage may result in a variety of abnormalities including sensineuronal deafness, vertigo and tinnitus. Myxoedematous infiltration of the eustachian tube may also produce signs of a conduction defect. There is no information on the relative importance of reversible deafness and irreversible presbyacusis in elderly hypothyroid patients. In association with diminished hearing, the elderly myxoedematous patient may have a characteristic husky voice or hoarseness.

Thyrotoxicosis may produce the characteristic eye changes of proptosis, exophthalmos, lid lag and lid retraction, but these are relatively uncommon in old age. Other more common disorders do, however, produce similar changes. For example, in chronic obstructive airways disease there may be proptosis. This, coupled with lid retraction due to sympathomimetic therapy, produces changes similar to those of thyrotoxic exophthalmos. Again muscle wasting may produce an appearance resembling that of lid lag.

Changes in the connective tissue of the skin modify interpretation of signs in the hands and forearms. For example, reduced elasticity means that it is extremely difficult to assess skin turgor and dehydration. The dermis may also be thin and tear with minimal injury. This is sometimes indicative of corticosteroid excess or ascorbic acid deficiency. Often, however, no cause can be found, so that this may be an extreme effect of ageing. Some gerontologists have suggested that, in old age, there is a link between a thin skin and bone rarefaction, but the evidence is far from convincing. In overt hypothyroidism the cool dry scaly slightly roughened skin is usually present in old people.

Extensive bruising may also be due to Cushing's syndrome or ascorbic acid deficiency. There is clear evidence, however, that bruising of the hands and forearms (senile purpura) is due to reduced skin and blood vessel elasticity (Shuster and Scarborough 1961). Shearing forces move the skin through a wide range of positions, so that friable blood vessels connecting the dermis with deeper layers are ruptured.

Thyroid Gland

It is important to look consciously for a thyroidectomy scar. A wrinkled skin and skeletal deformity may conceal this if only a cursory examination is made.

When palpating the thyroid, it is important to appreciate that ageing has a variety of effects. The first is that, in thyrotoxicosis, the gland is less likely to be palpable, and when there is enlargement this is more often nodular than diffuse. Even if the goitre is non-toxic it is more likely to be nodular than diffuse.

Thyroid cancer and lymphoma are more common in old age and should be considered if there is rapid enlargement of the gland, or if it feels hard and irregular or is attached to surrounding structures. Multinodular goitres are rarely malignant. A single nodule is more likely to be malignant, though this likelihood declines with increasing age. It is also important to assess carefully the lymph nodes in the neck for any evidence of enlargement.

Body Build

In both men and women, ageing is associated with an increase in the proportion of the body consisting of fat (Shepard 1978) (Fig. 2.3). This change is related to an increase in intra-abdominal fat and infiltration of skeletal muscle with fat while there is an actual decline in subcutaneous fat over the extremities.

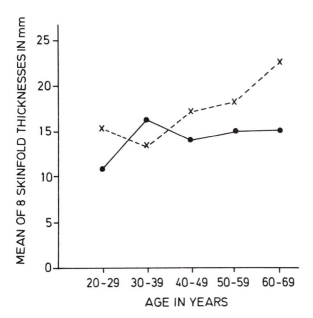

Fig. 2.3. Age and skinfold thickness in men (*solid circles*) and women (*crosses*). (After Shepard 1978.)

The simplest way of quantifying subcutaneous fat is to use Harpenden callipers to measure skinfold thickness over the mid-point of the left triceps. A more general picture of the proportion of body fat is given by measuring skinfold thicknesses over the triceps, biceps, subscapular and suprailiac areas calculating their sum, and from this using tables constructed by Durnin and Womersley (1974) to estimate percentage body fat.

A variety of endocrine disorders can cause obesity. In old people one of the more common is Cushing's syndrome due to corticosteroid therapy. This obesity characteristically affects the trunk, the face and the back of the neck, sparing the limbs. Cushing's syndrome due to other conditions and Cushing's disease are equally uncommon in old age as in other groups.

Obesity is also often associated with non-insulin-dependent diabetes in the elderly, where the obesity accentuates tissue insulin resistance.

Although hyperthyroidism is frequently associated with weight loss in old people, hypothyroidism is not an important cause for obesity in this group.

Cardiovascular System

Blood Pressure

Cross-sectional studies have established that there is a rise in blood pressure with increasing age (MacLennan 1986). The rise in systolic pressure is the more striking and continues until the age of 70, whereas that for the diastolic pressure is less marked and levels off over the age of 60. Longitudinal studies have confirmed that these changes also occur in individuals. However, environmental factors are probably involved in that age-related changes in blood pressure do not occur in isolated communities such as those in the Amazon Basin or South Sea Islands. Patients in long-stay mental institutions also have lower blood pressure than contemporaries in the community.

Although age has an important effect on blood pressure, a proportion of elderly patients have secondary hypertension. This is usually associated with renal disease, but endocrine disorders should also be considered. Though hyperaldosteronism only occurs in about 1% of patients with hypertension, it is found in all age groups. Phaeochromocytoma is extremely rare, occurring in only one out of 1000 hypertensive patients, but has a peak incidence between the ages of 50 and 69 (Sutton et al. 1981). A more common endocrine problem is hypertension due to treatment with corticosteroids.

Although hypertension is a problem in old people in general, it is less common in those attending a day hospital or requiring admission to a geriatric unit (Mac-Lennan 1986). Physical inactivity, poor cardiac function and electrolyte imbalance are all factors which contribute to this. If a disabled elderly person presents with hypotension and weight loss, there is the dilemma as to whether he should be investigated for adrenocortical insufficiency. In most instances, adrenal function is normal, and stimulation tests should be reserved for patients with buccal or flexural pigmentation or electrolyte abnormalities. Elderly patients with hypopituitarism usually present with pallor and postural hypotension (Belchetz 1985). Diagnosis is facilitated if serum thyroxine tests are performed routinely on frail elderly patients.

Peripheral Vascular Disease

The proportion of people with absent dorsalis pedis and posterior tibial pulses increases with age (Milne and Williamson 1972) (Fig. 2.4). Though many patients with this abnormality have no symptoms, an increased proportion have intermittent claudication, suggesting that absent pedal pulses are the result of atherosclerosis rather than physiological ageing. Pedal pulses also disappear in non-insulin-dependent diabetes, and the likelihood of this happening increases with the duration of disease (Kreines et al. 1985). This statistical association occurs independently from that of age and internal occlusion. The clinical relevance of this is that an elderly patient with diabetes has an extremely high risk of developing peripheral vascular disease which may manifest initially as ischaemic ulceration or digital gangrene.

Cardiac Disease

Ageing modifies the clinical presentation of hyperthyroidism so that the only manifestation may be that of cardiac disease (Davis and Davis 1974) (Table 2.4). The most common forms of this are atrial fibrillation and congestive cardiac failure. In old age, however, multiple pathology is the rule so that hyperthyroidism may coincide with coronary artery disease, chronic rheumatic heart disease, or other car-

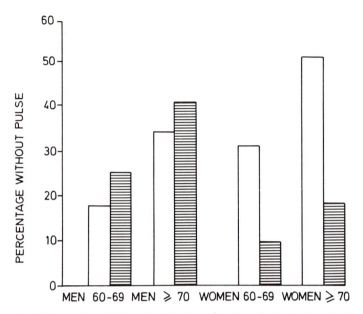

Fig. 2.4. Proportion of old people with absent dorsalis pedis (*hatched bars*) and posterior tibial pulses. (After Milne and Williamson 1972.)

Table 2.4. Cardiovascular manifestations of thyrotoxicosis in 85 patients over the age of 60 (Davis and Davis 1974)

Abnormality	Percentage prevalence
Tachycardia	58
Atrial fibrillation	39
Cardiomegaly	11
Systolic murmur	59
Hepatomegaly	45
Pitting oedema	50

diac disease. The only convincing evidence of cardiac disease being due to thyroid disease may be its response to antithyroid treatment.

Hypothyroidism accelerates the progression of coronary atherosclerosis. Usually, however, the problem only becomes apparent when replacement therapy increases the myocardial metabolism to induce angina, dysrhythmias, congestive cardiac failure or myocardial infarction. Hypothyroidism may also cause a pericardial effusion, although this is rarely of sufficient size to compromise cardiac function.

Diabetes mellitus increases cardiovascular morbidity and mortality by accelerating coronary atherosclerosis and occlusion (Mather et al. 1983). In addition, it may cause a cardiomyopathy associated with congestive cardiac failure.

Restrictive changes in the myocardium give rise to a thready pulse and a reduced or normal cardiac outline. There is debate as to whether the cardiomyopathy is primary or due to small vessel damage.

The high prevalence of cardiac disease in old people places them at particular risk from the mineralocorticoid effects of corticosteroids, such as sodium and water retention, hypokalaemia and hypertension. Fortunately, the mineralocorticoid effect of the synthetic steroids, prednisolone and prednisone, is slight and that of dexamethasone negligible. It is important, therefore, to look for alternative causes for cardiac failure in elderly patients on these latter drugs.

Urogenital System

Hormonal changes after the menopause result in the vaginal epithelium becoming atrophic (Studd and Thom 1981). Associated with this are secretory changes reducing vaginal acidity and leading to secondary infection so that the epithelium may be red and inflamed. Since the urethra and trigone have the same embryological origin as the vagina, their epithelium develops similar atrophic changes, resulting in frequency, nocturia, dysuria and even urinary incontinence. Therefore, in assessing the basis of these symptoms, vaginal examination may be useful in distinguishing atrophic urethritis from other causes such as cystitis, a lax pelvic floor or a hypertonic bladder.

A vaginal discharge and inflammation of the labia is often indicative of candidiasis, a common complication of diabetes mellitus. Indeed, this is often the presenting feature of type II diabetes in elderly women.

In elderly men there may be some testicular atrophy, but there is a great deal of individual variation, and if the process occurs at all it progresses very gradually (Davidson et al. 1983). Compared with changes in mental attitude and general health, testicular atrophy has minimal effects on sexual activity.

Over the age of 60 in men there is often a rapid increase in the size of the prostate gland. This results from a change in the relative concentrations of androgens and oestrogens, but the exact mechanism has not been elucidated yet.

Gastro-intestinal Tract

Despite popular folklore, ageing is not associated with a decline in colonic function. Constipation, however, is associated with a wide range of conditions common in old age including subnutrition, immobility, neurological disorders and depression. Hypothyroidism may also cause constipation, but in old people with multiple pathology its value as a discriminant symptom is lost.

A variety of endocrine disorders may cause diarrhoea. Diabetic autonomic neuropathy may cause bouts of diarrhoea which alternate with constipation. Hyperthyroidism may also cause diarrhoea, but the symptom is less common in the elderly. Diarrhoea and abdominal pain are classical features of Addison's disease, but the condition is so rare that it should only be considered if the symptoms are associated with other features such as buccal pigmentation, cachexia or electrolyte imbalance.

Locomotor System

Muscles

Ageing is associated with a decline in both muscle mass and muscle power (Mac-Lennan et al. 1980b) (Fig. 2.5). The process is mainly due to the death of anterior horn neurones. Initially, surviving neurones compensate for this by producing axon branches to renervate denervated muscle fibres. Eventually, however, there are insufficient surviving neurones to maintain the process. The clinical consequence is that muscle mass and power may be maintained late into old age when there is then a rapid decline in function. Physical activity also is important, so that the individuals who maintain this in old age retain a higher level of muscle function. An adequate protein intake is also crucial to maintaining muscle mass. This is a particular problem in sick old people, where anorexia and increased catabolism combine to cause gross muscle wasting.

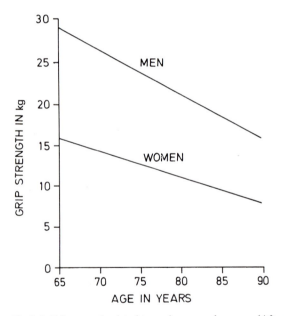

Fig. 2.5. Grip strength related to age in men and women. (After MacLennan et al. 1980b.)

A further factor confounding the evaluation of endocrine disease as a cause of muscle weakness is the wide range of disorders which interfere with limb function. These include osteoarthritis, Parkinsonism and cerebrovascular disease.

Muscle weakness is common in thyroid disease. In hypothyroidism there is hypertrophy of type I muscle fibres, but atrophy of type II ones, so that the overall picture is that of muscle weakness, with no atrophy or with hypertrophy (Khaleeli et al. 1983b). Associated features include muscle cramps, muscle stiffness and sluggish tendon reflexes.

Proximal muscle atrophy and weakness is common in hyperthyroidism occurring to some degree in around 80% of patients (Tajima et al. 1984). Unlike other myopathies, the tendon reflexes are increased and brisk. The histological picture is that of generalised fibre atrophy with fat cell infiltration.

Both Cushing's syndrome and corticosteroid therapy are associated with wasting and weakness of proximal muscles (Khaleeli et al. 1983a). Involvement of the quadriceps group makes it difficult to climb stairs or to rise from a squatting position and produces a characteristic waddling gait. Marked myopathy and hypokalaemia are common when Cushing's syndrome is due to ectopic production of ACTH by a malignant tumour.

Patients with vitamin D deficiency present with similar signs (Schott and Wills 1976). The myopathy is unrelated to hypocalcaemia, but is a direct effect of either 25-hydroxyvitamin D or 1,25-dihydroxyvitamin D deficiency. Since both immobility and vitamin D deficiency are common in old people it is difficult to establish whether the two are directly related to each other. Indeed, since immobility results in reduced sunlight exposure with a decline in calciferol synthesis, it is often difficult to distinguish cause from effect.

Diabetes mellitus has a variety of effects on muscle function. An example is that elderly diabetics complain of cramps. However, there have been no definitive studies to establish whether they are more common in diabetics than in old people in general. Another manifestation is muscle wasting of the hands and feet associated with a motor neuropathy (Borsey et al. 1983). The condition is much less common than a sensory neuropathy with a prevalence of around 1.8 per 1000 diabetics, and usually develops 10–20 years after the onset of the condition. In the elderly, the condition is easily mistaken for the effects of ageing on the small muscles of the hands. Again, quadriceps weakness, often asymmetrical, may be the result of diabetic amyotrophy (Choknovesty et al. 1977). Other features of this include muscle pains, fasciculation and absent tendon reflexes. These signs are often wrongly attributed to age and non-specific disability.

Occasionally, old people develop severe hypokalaemia, and present with profound general muscle weakness. This is usually the result of diuretic therapy but occasionally follows ectopic secretion of adrenocorticotrophic hormones. There is more doubt as to whether the more common problem of mild potassium depletion in the elderly associated with dietary deficiency and diuretic therapy has an effect on muscle power (MacLennan 1981). Different studies have yielded conflicting results; so for the present, it is reasonable to assume that, if a patient has a normal serum potassium concentration, treatment with potassium supplements will have no effect upon muscle power.

Skeleton

The most important clinical consequence of bone rarefaction is an increasing incidence of fractures of the proximal femur, the pelvis, the neck of humerus and the distal forearm (Paterson and MacLennan 1984). Crush fractures of vertebral bodies give rise to severe back pain accompanied by an increasing kyphosis.

Bone rarefaction is a natural concomitant of ageing and usually commences in early middle age. It affects both sexes, but there are particularly striking changes in women immediately after the menopause.

A variety of endocrine problems accelerate the process, but the one of most practical clinical importance is corticosteroid excess. This inhibits both collagen synthesis by osteoblasts, and calcium absorption from the gut, and manifests itself as a crush fracture of a vertebrae or a fractured proximal femur. The risk is compounded if corticosteroids are used in elderly women with rheumatoid arthritis, a condition also associated with osteoporosis.

Hyperthyroidism promotes bone rarefaction by stimulating osteoclastic activity. Cases of elderly hyperthyroid patients sustaining fractures have been reported, but the problem is uncommon, and negligible compared with the risk of hyperthyroidism precipitating cardiac disease.

There is considerable controversy over the effect of diabetes mellitus on bone mass. It would appear that longstanding insulin-dependent diabetes normally leads to some degree of bone rarefaction. The effect in non-insulin-dependent diabetes is more varied with most obese patients in this group having an increased rather than a decreased bone mass. As a consequence, diabetes-induced osteoporosis is rarely a problem in the elderly.

The increasing use of automated biochemical analysis in hospitals has increased the frequency with which hypercalcaemia due to primary hyperparathyroidism has been identified. It occurs occasionally in elderly men, but is particularly prevalent in elderly women. Usually the condition is asymptomatic, but some patients go on to exhibit the systemic effects of hypercalcaemia. A few also have radiological evidence of bone resorption, but this is rare, and clinical complications of this even rarer.

Peripheral Nerves

With increasing age there is a decline in both position sense and vibration sense (MacLennan et al. 1980c) (Fig. 2.6) (Table 2.5). There also are changes in touch, pain and temperature sense, but these are more difficult to quantify. In addition, if standard techniques are used, the proportion of individuals with absent ankle reflexes increases with age (Table 2.5). The pathological basis for these changes is uncertain, but they suggest peripheral nerve degeneration resulting from either primary degeneration or obstruction of the vasae nervorum.

Diabetes mellitus also causes peripheral nerve degeneration. Age-related changes make it extremely difficult to evaluate this in the elderly. Sensory symptoms such as cramps, coldness, deadness and tingling are relatively common, so that even these may not give a clue to the presence of a neuropathy. One of the most characteristic features is an unpleasant burning sensation in the feet, occurring particularly at night and causing the patient to throw the bedclothes off his legs. The most serious consequence of the disorder is that sensory loss, coupled with macro- and microvascular changes, leads to ulceration and infection of the foot. Careful examination is essential in detecting early changes, in that a small, apparently superficial lesion may cover an existing underlying area of necrosis or a collar stud abscess. Corns, bunions and even neglected toenails should be identified to ensure treatment by an experienced chiropodist.

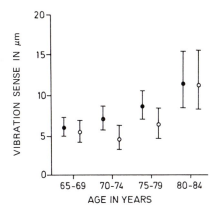

Fig. 2.6. Effect of age on knee vibratory threshold in men (*solid circles*) and women (*open circles*). Bars indicate 95% confidence limits of the mean. (After MacLennan et al. 1980c.)

Table 2.5. Effects of age on position sense and ankle reflexes (MacLennan et al. 1980c)

Age (years)	Percentage absent position sense		Percentage absent ankle reflexes	
	Men	Women	Men	Women
65–69	4.7	14.7	4.5	6.1
70–74	12.7	13.8	6.3	4.0
75–79	35.0	46.3	19.5	14.3
80–84	45.8	41.2	15.8	23.1

Apart from the motor and sensory changes already described, diabetes may be associated with damage to single nerves resulting in peroneal nerve palsy, sciatica or oculomotor palsy in addition to median and ulnar nerve compression syndromes (Fraser et al. 1979). Since these disorders are asymmetrical and are not a normal feature of ageing, they should be more easily identified.

Myxoedema gives rise to a variety of peripheral nerve lesions. The most common is paraesthesia of the fingers usually associated with median nerve compression in the carpal tunnel. Other nerve entrapment syndromes occur but are less common. A true peripheral neuropathy has been described but is rarer. Again, hypothyroidism is sometimes associated with cerebellar degeneration, so that the condition is an occasional cause of ataxia and falls in the elderly.

Autonomic Dysfunction

Ageing is associated with a decline in the function of the autonomic nervous system. Manifestations of a deterioration in the parasympathetic nervous system include decreased variation in beat-to-beat intervals on deep respiration, reduced

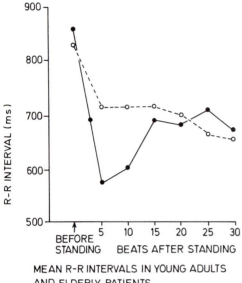

MEAN R-R INTERVALS IN YOUNG ADULTS
AND ELDERLY PATIENTS

Fig. 2.7. Heart rate response to standing in young (*solid circles*) and elderly (*open circles*) subjects.
(After MacLennan and Ritch 1979.)

prolongation of beat-to-beat intervals in the expiratory phase of the Valsalva manoeuvre, and impairment of the bradycardia response on standing (MacLennan
and Ritch 1979) (Fig. 2.7).

Evidence of sympathetic degeneration is less convincing (MacLennan et al.
1980a). Postural hypotension is common in old age, but other tests of sympathetic
function such as the diastolic blood pressure response to sustained grip strength
are unimpaired. It seems likely, therefore, that in old age, postural hypotension
may be the result of reduced vascular compliance.

A proportion of patients with longstanding diabetes exhibit signs of autonomic
degeneration (Ewing and Clarke 1982). In the elderly, however, it is almost
impossible to separate the effects of diabetes on cardiovascular regulation from
those of ageing. The effects of diabetes on bladder function are more relevant, in
that apart from drug therapy, diabetes is the most common cause of an atonic
bladder in the elderly. Parkinson's disease is another occasional cause while tabes
dorsalis is now rare.

Infections

Ageing is associated with a decline in both lymphocyte-mediated immunological
reactions and in neutrophil polymorphonuclear leucocyte chemotaxis (Fox 1984).
There is no consistent change in antibody production. The clinical consequences
are that old people are more susceptible to infections, and that clinical manifesta-

tions such as pyrexia, leucocytes and localising signs are less obvious.

Poor control of diabetes mellitus produces impairment in both neutrophil and lymphocyte function, so that patients show increased susceptibility to infection, and suffer more severe infection (Son and Lauria 1983). Those causing particular problems include candidiasis of the skin and mucosal surfaces, bacterial infections of the skin and subcutaneous tissues, urinary tract infections, bacteraemia, infection of foot ulcers, bronchopneumonia and tuberculosis. The diagnosis of these is particularly difficult in diabetic ketoacidosis or hyperglycaemic hyperosmolar coma, where electrolyte imbalance and hypothermia suppress the normal manifestations of infection.

Corticosteroids increase the risk and local spread of infection by inhibiting the tissue response and antibody formation in infection. Problems include the reactivation of tuberculosis and masking of the clinical signs of an infection. Mucocutaneous fungal infections are also common.

References

American College of Physicians. Health and Public Policy Committee (1984) The dexamethasone suppression test for detection, diagnosis and management of depression. Ann Intern Med 100: 307–308

Belchetz P (1985) Idiopathic hypopituitarism in the elderly. Br Med J 291: 247–248

Borsey DQ, Cull RE, Fraser DM et al. (1983) Generalised small muscle wasting of the hands in diabetes mellitus. Diabetes Care 6: 10–17

Carroll BJ, Feinberg M, Greden JF et al. (1981) A specific laboratory test for the diagnosis of melancholia. Arch Gen Psychiatry 138: 15–22

Choknovesty S, Royes MG, Rubina FA, Tonalei H (1977) The syndrome of diabetic amyotrophy. Ann Neurol 2: 181–194

Davidson JM, Chen JJ, Crapo L et al. (1983) Hormonal changes and sexual function in ageing men. J Clin Endocrinol Metab 57: 71–77

Davis PJ, Davis FB (1974) Hyperthyroidism in patients over the age of 60 years. Clinical features in 85 patients. Medicine 53: 161–181

Durnin JVGA, Womersley J (1974) Body fat assessed from total body density and its estimation from skinfold thickness measurements on 481 men and women from 16–77 years. Br J Nutr 32: 77–79

Ewing DJ, Clarke BF (1982) Diagnosis and management of diabetic autonomic neuropathy. Br Med J 285: 916–918

Forester CP (1963) Coma in myxoedema. Arch Intern Med 111: 700–743

Fox RA (1984) Immunology and infection in the elderly. Churchill Livingstone, London

Fraser DM, Campbell IWC, Ewing DJ, Clarke BF (1979) Mononeuropathy in diabetes mellitus. Diabetes 28: 96–101

Heldeman JH, Elahi D, Anderson DK et al. (1983) Prevention of the glucose intolerance of thiazide diuretics by maintenance of body potassium. Diabetes 32: 106–111

Khaleeli AA, Edwards RHT, Gohil K et al. (1983a) Corticosteroid myopathy: a clinical and pathological study. Clin Endocrinol 18: 155–166

Khaleeli AA, Griffith DG, Edwards RHT (1983b) The clinical presentation of hypothyroid myopathy and its relationship to abnormalities in structure and function of skeletal muscle. Clin Endocrinol 19: 365–376

Kreines K, Johnson E, Albrink M et al. (1985) The course of peripheral vascular disease in non-insulin dependent diabetes. Diabetes Care 8: 235–243

Ling MHM, Perry PJ, Tsuang MT (1981) Side effects of corticosteroid therapy–psychiatric aspects. Arch Gen Psychiatry 38: 471–477

MacLennan WJ (1981) The problem of potassium. In: Caird FI, Evans JG (eds) Advanced geriatric medicine 1. Pitman, London, pp 67–72

MacLennan WJ (1985) Hypothermia. In: Lye MD (ed) Acute geriatric medicine. MTP Press, pp 75–92

MacLennan WJ (1986) Epidemiology of hypertension. In: Advanced geriatric medicine 5. Pitman, London, pp 79–88

MacLennan WJ, Ritch AES (1979) Heart-rate response to standing as a test for autonomic neuropathy. Br Med J 1: 505

MacLennan WJ, Martin P, Mason BJ (1975) Energy intake, disability, disease and skinfold thickness in a long stay hospital. Gerontol Clin 17: 173–180

MacLennan WJ, Hall MRP, Timothy JI (1980a) Postural hypotension in old age: is it a disorder of the nervous system or of blood vessels? Age Ageing 9: 25–32

MacLennan WJ, Hall MRP, Timothy J, Robinson M (1980b) Is weakness in old age due to muscle wasting? Age Ageing 9: 188–192

MacLennan WJ, Timothy JI, Hall MRP (1980c) Vibration sense, proprioception and ankle reflexes in old age. J Clin Exp Gerontol 2: 159–172

Mather SR, Garber AJ, Atter M et al. (1983) Managing cardiac disease in patients with diabetes mellitus. Geriatrics 38: 81–90

Milne JS, Williamson J (1972) Intermittent claudication and peripheral pulses in older people. Age Ageing 1: 146–151

Paterson CR, MacLennan WJ (1984) Bone disease in the elderly. John Wiley, Chichester

Schott GD, Wills MR (1976) Muscle weakness in osteomalacia. Lancet 1, 626–629

Shepard RJ (1978) Physical fitness and ageing. Croom Helm, London.

Shuster S, Scarborough LH (1961) Senile purpura. Q J Med 54: 33–40

Son P, Lauria DB (1983) Infectious complications in the elderly diabetic. Geriatrics 38: 63–72

Studd JWW, Thom MH (1981) Ovarian failure and ageing. Clin Endocrinol Metab 10: 89–113

Sutton MG, Sheps SG, Lie JT (1981) Prevalence of clinically unsuspected phaeochromocytoma – a review of a 50 year autopsy series. Mayo Clin Proc 56: 354–360

Tajima K, Mashita K, Yamone T et al. (1984) Thyrotoxic myopathy associated with subacute thyroiditis. Clin Endocrinol 20: 307–312

Thomas B, Mazzaferri EL, Skillman TG (1970) Apathetic thyrotoxicosis: a distinctive clinical and laboratory entity. Ann Intern Med 72: 679–685

Tomlinson BE, Blessed G, Roth M (1970) Observations on the brains of demented old people. J Neurol Sci 11: 205–242

Wenzel KW (1981) Pharmacological interference with in vitro tests of thyroid function. Metabolism 30: 717–732

Wilkinson DG (1981) Psychiatric aspects of diabetes mellitus. Br J Psychiatry 138: 1–9

3 Thyroid Disease

Thyroid disease is an important and relatively common cause of mental and physical morbidity. Since treatment is usually relatively simple, and often effective in reducing disability, it is important that the condition should not be missed. In old age, unfortunately, the signs and symptoms of thyroid disease are masked so that reliance cannot be placed on clinical judgement alone, and all elderly people showing signs of recent but gradual mental or physical deterioration should be investigated for laboratory evidence of thyroid disease. This is one of the few situations in which there is justification for laboratory screening in the elderly (Hodkinson and Denham 1977).

Investigation of Suspected Thyroid Disease

Strategies for the laboratory investigation of suspected thyroid disease are outlined in Chap. 12. Increasingly, laboratories are performing a highly sensitive thyroid stimulating hormone (TSH) assay as a first line test of thyroid function. If this is normal (and provided that the patient is not being assessed for hypothalamic-pituitary disease) then the patient is generally euthyroid. If the TSH is suppressed, this suggests that the patient may be hyperthyroid and this may be confirmed by assay of the serum free or total thyroxine (fT_4 or TT_4) and if necessary, serum free or total tri-iodothyronine (fT_3 or TT_3) concentrations. An elevated TSH is indicative of primary hypothyroidism and this can be confirmed by a low serum fT_4 or TT_4 level.

Changes due to Ageing

In healthy old people, serum T_4 and thyroxine binding globulin (TBG) levels are similar to those found in young and middle-aged adults (Caplan et al. 1981). There is a decline in serum TT_3 levels however (Table 3.1). An increased proportion of

Table 3.1. Age and serum total triiodothyronine (TT3) concentrations (Caplan et al. 1981)

| Age (years) | Serum T_3 (ng/dl) | |
	Mean	95% confidence limits
16–24	133	91–175
65–74	119	75–163
75–84	103	55–151
85–100	93	51–135

old people (with normal serum T_4) have elevated serum TSH levels, around 20% having levels over 5 mU/l and 6% values over 10 mU/l (Sawin et al. 1979). Despite this change, it is reasonable to assume that an elderly patient with a low serum thyroxine and a TSH of over 5 mU/l has primary hypothyroidism.

Effect of Illness

A wide range of disorders common in old age have a striking effect on thyroid function tests. These effects have received considerable attention of late and are commonly referred to as being due to non-thyroidal illness (NTI) or the sick euthyroid syndrome. The end result is a low serum total T_3 concentration. In NTI the serum of patients contains substances possibly oleic and other free fatty acids, which are released from tissues and inhibit the conversion of T_4 to T_3 (Chopra et al. 1985) while reverse T_3 is increased. These inhibitors also appear to affect the binding of thyroid hormones to binding sites on their binding proteins and may also affect uptake of thyroid hormones into cells (Chopra et al. 1985).

Complex combinations of these factors mean that though TT_3 is always low in NTI, TT_4 can be high, normal or low. Free thyroid hormone levels measured by equilibrium dialysis are also variable, while fT_4 and fT_3 measured by other methods are often low and probably meaningless. Where NTI is particularly severe there may be a hypothalamic-pituitary defect with reduced levels of TSH. These common abnormalities of thyroid function settle spontaneously as the clinical condition improves.

A low T_3 syndrome in an acute intercurrent illness makes it difficult to confirm a suspected diagnosis of hyperthyroidism, and there are case reports where, when a patient has recovered from an acute illness, TT_3 concentrations have risen into the hyperthyroid range. This means that if a patient with severe NTI is suspected of being hyperthyroid, a serum TT_3 level above 1 mmol/l should be considered as highly suspicious of hyperthyroidism.

The stress of psychiatric illness may also modify thyroid function tests (Levy et al. 1981). Both total and free serum T_4 levels may be elevated, returning to normal when mental symptoms are controlled. In this situation the serum T_3 is usually normal. Less commonly the serum T_4 and T_3 levels are reduced although the serum TSH level is normal. These changes in general psychiatric populations require more detailed evaluation in elderly patients with acute confusional states, dementia or depression. Observations of elevated thyroid hormone levels during acute psychiatric illness have major implications for the routine screening of psychiatric patients on admission to a mental hospital.

A wide range of drugs may affect conventional thyroid function tests by altering the serum TBG concentration; decreasing by competitive inhibition the T_4 or T_3 uptake by thyroid hormone binding proteins; induction of T_4 and T_3 metabolism; inhibition of T_4 conversion to T_3; or inhibition of thyroid function (Wenzel 1981) (Table 3.2). This is of particular relevance in old age when polypharmacy associated with multiple pathology is common. There is as yet little experience on the impact of the newer thyroid function test strategies on these drug induced problems, particularly those due to binding inhibitions. In general a sensitive TSH assay should be a satisfactory test for euthyroidism in these circumstances, but problems might arise where drugs have specific effects on thyrotrophin secretion by the pituitary.

Table 3.2. Drugs commonly used in old people which produce changes in thyroid function (Wenzel 1981)

Drug	Effect	Mode of action
Oestrogen	↑ T_4	Increased binding activity
Stanazolol	↓ T_4	Decreased binding capacity
Salicylates	↓ T_4	Competitive binding of transport protein
	↓ T_3	Competitive binding of transport protein
Heparin	↓ T_4	Competitive binding of transport protein
Diazepam	↓ T_4	Competitive binding of transport protein
Sulphonylureas	↓ T_4	Competitive binding of transport protein
Carbamazepine	↓ T_4	Enzyme induction
	↓ T_3	Enzyme induction
Phenytoin	↓ T_3	Unknown
	↓ T_3	Unknown
Propranolol	↓ T_3	Inhibition of T_4 conversion
Co-trimoxazole	↓ T_4	Thyroidal inhibition
	↓ T_3	Thyroidal inhibition
Iodides	↓ T_4	Thyroidal inhibition
	↓ T_3	Thyroidal inhibition
Thiazides	↑ T_3	Change in volume of distribution
Phenothiazines	↓ T_4	Unknown

Hypothyroidism

Hypothyroidism is 14 times as common in women as men, and in the former has an overall prevalence in the community of around 2% (Tunbridge et al. 1977). A recent large community survey of women over the age of 60 produced a similar prevalence rate of 1.87%, in which 0.55% had previously undetected hypothyroidism (Falkenberg et al. 1983). In a review of elderly women admitted to hospital the prevalence was higher at 3.9% with 2.9% of the total having previously undetected disease (Bahemuka and Hodkinson 1975). A practical implication of this is that, in the community, it would be necessary to perform 200 screening tests to identify one elderly woman with unidentified hypothyroidism, whereas 33 tests would achieve this in elderly women admitted to hospital. The prevalence of the disease is so much lower in men that it is difficult to justify screening under any circumstances, and testing should be reserved for those with clinical pointers to thyroid disease.

Pathogenesis

The most common cause of hypothyroidism in old age is auto-immune thyroiditis characterised by lymphocyte and plasma cell infiltration of the thyroid gland with fibrosis and destruction of follicles. A wide range of auto-antibodies have been detected in the serum of up to 80% of patients, but those of most diagnostic value are thyroglobulin (TGHA) and microsomal (MCHA) haemagglutinating anti-bodies (Doniach et al. 1979). While ageing has no effect on the prevalence of these in men, both antibodies are more common in women and show a striking increase with age (Tunbridge et al. 1977). Auto-immune thyroiditis represents a range of disorders from so called Hashimoto's thyroiditis (often euthyroid with diffuse firm thyroid enlargement) to primary thyroid atrophy (usually hypothyroid with no palpable goitre). Ageing is associated with a decline in the proportion of women with auto-immune thyroiditis who have a palpable or visible thyroid gland.

Hypothyroidism in old people may also be the result of treatment of hyper-thyroidism with radio-iodine (^{131}I). Standard doses produce a cumulative increase in the incidence of hypothyroidism so that by 10 years around 70% suffer from the

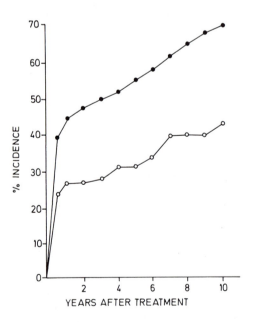

Fig. 3.1. Cumulative percentage increase of hypothyroidism in patients treated with ^{131}I (*solid circles*) and surgery (*open circles*) for thyrotoxicosis. (After Nofal et al. 1966.)

condition (Nofal et al. 1966) (Fig. 3.1). The problem is particularly prevalent in old age since ^{131}I therapy is reserved for the treatment of thyrotoxicosis beyond childbearing age, and the cumulative incidence of hypothyroidism continues to increase indefinitely into extreme old age. This emphasises the crucial importance of adequate follow up of patients treated with radio-iodine, even if mental or physical incapacity make this difficult.

The incidence of hypothyroidism is lower after partial thyroidectomy than after ^{131}I therapy, but even here there is a progressive increase in the cumulative frequency of the condition so that by 10 years after surgery over 40% of patients are hypothyroid (Nofal et al. 1966) (Fig. 3.1). It also appears that the natural history of hyperthyroid Graves' disease is such that, even without radiotherapy or surgery, a significant proportion of patients eventually progress to thyroid atrophy and hypothyroidism.

In a few instances hypothyroidism in old age is due to hypopituitarism (Chap. 8). Other rare causes of hypothyroidism in an elderly person are painless thyroiditis, neoplastic destruction of the gland (e.g. by lymphoma), Reidel's thyroiditis and drug ingestion (e.g. amiadorone).

Clinical Features

The myriad ways in which hypothyroidism presents in the elderly is discussed in Chap. 2. Characteristically, the signs in old age develop insidiously, are ill defined and are atypical. In view of this it is essential that thyroid function tests should be arranged if there is the slightest suspicion that a patient may be hypothyroid.

Attempts to refine the clinical assessment of hypothyroidism in the elderly have had limited success. Indices of scores for symptoms and signs are useless. The only test of value is the ankle reflex (Cropper 1973). Measurement with a photomotograph quantifies specific slowing of the relaxation phase of the reflex. An obvious limitation is that the test can only be performed if the patient has an ankle reflex. Other tendon reflexes are affected, but these is no simple way of quantifying these.

Subclinical Hypothyroidism

In this condition, the patient has no or non-specific complaints related to thyroid dysfunction, and appears clinically euthyroid. There may have been previous therapy for hyperthyroidism or there may be underlying auto-immune thyroiditis with goitre. The serum TT_4 concentration is usually below or in the lower part of the normal range, while the serum TT_3 level is usually well maintained by an elevated serum TSH. If there are high circulating levels of thyroid auto-antibodies there is a significant risk of progression to frank hypothyroidism (5% per annum) (Tunbridge et al. 1977).

Whether this condition should be treated is controversial. Controlled trials of thyroxine replacement therapy in younger patients with this condition have shown no significant benefit (Ridgeway et al. 1981; Bell et al. 1985). The case for treating elderly patients with this condition has not been satisfactorily addressed.

Myxoedema Coma

This is a state of severe hypothyroidism in which a patient has become drowsy or unconscious. The condition carries a grave prognosis and is particularly prone to occur in elderly women during the winter. In a review of 77 cases of myxoedema coma, all showed facial changes characteristic of hypothyroidism, although it could be that this resulted from the diagnosis only being made in patients with typical features (Forrester 1963). Patients may be hypotensive, are usually areflexic and may convulse. Other features are those of coma and hypothermia. The coma may be the result of several factors with a reduced cerebral blood flow, hypoxia, hypercapnia, hyponatraemia and sedative drugs all contributing.

In clinical practice the difficulty is that of distinguishing hypothermia due to hypothyroidism from that due to other causes. If the patient shows typical facial features, it is likely that she will receive appropriate treatment, but if she does not she will probably die with the condition unrecognised. Serum creatinine phosphokinase levels may be markedly elevated representing release of the enzyme from severely myxoedematous (sometimes traumatised) muscle. In the past, thyroid function tests in the acute situation have been of little value since they have usually provided only retrospective information. There has also been the problem of distinguishing hypothyroidism from non-thyroidal illness. Newer strategies of thyroid function testing with the use of sensitive TSH assays as the first line thyroid function test may provide a definitive answer much more quickly.

Treatment

There has been no satisfactory study on the most appropriate dose of L-thyroxine for initiating therapy in an elderly patient with hypothyroidism. Lean body mass is one of the determinants of the maintenance dose of thyroxine so that elderly subjects tend to require lower maintenance doses than younger subjects (Sawin et al. 1983), the usual dose being in the range of 50–150 µg daily (Rosenbaum and Bazel 1982). Patients often develop hypothyroidism insidiously and should be rendered euthyroid gradually. This is particularly important in patients who may have ischaemic heart disease in whom replacement thyroxine therapy can precipitate atrial fibrillation, heart failure or myocardial infarction or exacerbate angina.

Accordingly, with elderly subjects it may be wise to initiate L-thyroxine therapy at a dose of 25 µg daily. In patients with clinical or electrocardiographic evidence of ischaemic heart disease, the initial dose should be 25 µg on alternate days and if there is no contra-indication the patient should also receive a beta-adrenoceptor blocker to protect the heart from the increased workload induced by thyroid hormones.

The dose of L-thyroxine can then be gradually increased at approximately 4-weekly intervals until a satisfactory maintenance dose is achieved.

If treatment is being initiated for secondary hypothyroidism replacement hydrocortisone therapy must first be given to prevent thyroxine precipitating a hypoadrenal crisis.

If hyperthyroidism is treated with an ablative dose of ^{131}I and there is a rapid onset of hypothyroidism, the rapid change induces severe symptoms of hypothyroidism. This calls for an initial dose of thyroxine of 50 µg daily which may be increased after 2–4 weeks depending upon the clinical response.

Monitoring of Replacement Thyroxine Therapy

Biochemical monitoring of thyroxine replacement therapy is complex and is bedevilled by the lack of any reliable index of tissue thyroid status. Initially, the TRH test became the gold standard and it was thought that a suppressed TSH response to TRH (equivalent to an undetectable sensitive TSH using new methodology), represented over treatment with thyroxine (Evered et al. 1973). However, it became clear that if the thyroxine dosage was increased the peripheral conversion of T_4 to T_3 decreased so that the T_3 to T_4 ratio decreased. The elevated serum T_4, associated with this did not produce clinical signs of hyperthyroidism (McPherson et al. 1982). These supervened only if the serum T_3 became elevated (Rendell and Salmon 1985). In this situation the serum TSH was suppressed without elevation of serum fT_4 or fT_3 levels and without clinical evidence of hyperthyroidism (Mardell et al. 1985).

What can be confidently stated is that if patients on replacement therapy with thyroxine have elevated serum TSH concentrations, they are either on too small a dose or are poorly compliant with therapy. It is more difficult to detect over replacement. The diagnosis is primarily made on clinical grounds, when the TSH level is suppressed and the serum TT_3 or fT_3 concentration is increased (Pearce and Himsworth 1982).

A recent review of the various biochemical indices of thyroid function available concluded that these tests were of little value in monitoring patients receiving thyroxine replacement (Fraser et al. 1986). Our view is that clinical assessment of thyroxine replacement is important, and that sensitive tests of thyroid function such as TSH and fT_3 levels are useful adjuncts to the clinical evaluation. It would seem sensible to aim for a serum free T_3 in the normal range and a detectable but normal serum TSH.

Myxoedema Coma

There is no generally agreed plan of management for this disorder, particularly in respect to thyroid hormone replacement (Hurley 1983). Thus some authorities recommend initial treatment with a 500 µg intravenous bolus of L-thyroxine. Others recommend the administration of modest doses of T_4 (50 µg once daily) and T_3 (5 µg twice daily) via a nasogastric tube (Hall et al. 1980). Higher doses of T_3 (an initial bolus of 100 µg intravenously followed by 20 µg three times a day) have also been recommended (Toft et al. 1981).

Hypothermia associated with myxoedema should be treated in the standard fashion of gradual rewarming, administration of antibiotics and the management of any other intercurrent or complicating illness (MacLennan 1985). Patients suspected of having myxoedema coma are usually also given hydrocortisone initially 100 mg three times daily intravenously in case there is associated pituitary-adrenal failure because of hypopituitarism.

Despite full intensive care measures, including the use of assisted respiration, if necessary, the mortality rate is in excess of 50%, reflecting the advanced age and the severity of the presenting illness in these patients (Hylander and Rosenqvist 1985).

Hyperthyroidism

Prevalence

Hyperthyroidism is 5–12 times as common in women as in men (Tunbridge et al. 1977). In both sexes there is a striking increase in the incidence of new cases with age. Expressed as a prevalence, 1.9% of women over the age of 60 are thyrotoxic (Falkenberg et al. 1983). That for women admitted to a geriatric unit was 1.5% (Jeffreys 1972). In a consecutive series of 594 cases of hyperthyroidism, just over 10% were aged 70 years or older (Greenwood et al. 1985).

Causes

Whereas, in young patients, Graves' disease with diffuse toxic goitre is the most common cause of hyperthyroidism, this is not the case in older patients. In a group of hyperthyroid patients aged 70 years or older, half had no palpable goitre, 30% had nodular goitres (multiple or single) and 20% diffuse goitres. The majority with impalpable glands had positive antithyroid antibodies, and diffuse isotope uptake on thyroid scans, suggesting that they had underlying hyperthyroid Graves' disease (Greenwood et al. 1985). There also is considerable geographical variation in the frequency of toxic nodular goitre, in that it is more common as a cause of hyperthyroidism in young and elderly subjects in relatively iodine deficient areas such as Switzerland (Studer et al. 1985).

While Graves' disease and toxic nodular goitre account for the vast majority of new cases of hyperthyroidism in elderly patients, a small proportion have hyperthyroidism associated with a low thyroidal uptake of radio-iodine tracer (Himsworth 1985). This includes patients with iodine-induced hyperthyroidism, amiodarone-induced hyperthyroidism, those with various forms of thyroiditis, including sub-acute or deQuervain thyroiditis, painless thyroiditis (so-called Hashitoxicosis associated with auto-immune thyroiditis) and those with hyperthyroidism from excessive thyroid hormone administration (particularly of a thyroid extract containing T_3 and T_4).

Pathogenesis

In Graves' disease there is evidence of humoral- and cell-mediated auto-immunity against thyroid tissues. Of particular importance is the production of antibodies, usually of the IGG class, which are capable of causing activation of TSH receptors on thyroid follicular cells and hence causing chronic hyperstimulation of production and secretion of thyroid hormones. Various methods are available for the measurement of these antibodies, so that their nomenclature varies. An example is that, in one assay, antibodies are detected by their ability to inhibit the binding of TSH to its receptor and thus are known as TSH receptor-binding inhibitory immunoglobulins (TBII). Alternatively, the antibodies may be detected by their ability to stimulate thyroid slices in vitro and are known as thyroid-stimulating immunoglobulins (TSI).

Antibodies are detected in up to 80% of sera of patients with Graves' disease but it should be noted that the antibodies are heterogeneous and that serum with TBII activity may not necessarily have TSI activity. There is a high prevalence of other thyroid auto-antibodies in hyperthyroid patients but in elderly women their significance is unclear in that old people with toxic nodular goitres also have a high prevalance of microsomal antibodies (Greenwood et al. 1985).

The subject of toxic nodular goitre and its pathogenesis has recently been reviewed by Studer and colleagues (Studer et al. 1985). Patients with this usually have had long-standing goitres and indeed may have been treated with iodine for goitre in adolescence. Thyroid enlargement is slow and often unnoticed by the patient, but as this happens, follicles within the gland become autonomous in terms of thyroid hormone production so that they escape from TSH control. Excess thyroid hormone production may not initially be sufficient to cause hyperthyroidism but is sufficient to suppress TSH secretion and abolish the TSH response to intravenous TRH. Eventually hyperthyroidism gradually supervenes.

In this condition, palpation usually reveals multiple nodules and, even if one nodule is dominant, the rest of the gland is enlarged. The nodular pattern is related to the fibrosis and scarring consequent on necrosis of nodules whose growth has outgrown their blood supply. The cause of follicular growth is unclear but is not dependent on TSH. Immunoglobulins which stimulate thyroid follicular cells in vitro have been isolated from the sera of patients, and it may be that toxic nodular goitre is a separate form of immunologically mediated thyroid disease.

On thyroid scanning, palpable nodules are not necessarily functional. Conversely, functional areas on the scan may not correspond to palpable nodules. Indeed, autoradiographs of nodular goitres often show heterogeneity of function between follicles with considerable functional activity in follicular tissue between nodules.

A solitary toxic nodular adenoma is usually classified separately from toxic multi-nodular goitre. This is reasonable in younger patients where there is a hyperfunctioning nodule causing hyperthyroidism. While iodine uptake in the rest of the gland is suppressed, it can be stimulated by a TSH injection. This pattern is rare in the toxic solitary nodule of older patients where the condition should usually be considered as a variant of toxic multi-nodular goitre (Studer et al. 1985).

In the past, iodine-induced hyperthyroidism (IIH) was thought to be confined to patients with underlying thyroid pathology where iodine deficiency gave rise to a multinodular goitre which became toxic when the iodine intake was increased (Vagenakis et al. 1972; Stewart and Vidor 1976). IIH has been identified more recently in patients with normal thyroid glands. In one series, 67 out of 85 patients had no underlying thyroid disorder and 43 of them were on treatment with amiodarone (Leger et al. 1984). The use of amiodarone in older patients with dysrhythmias is steadily increasing. The drug contains 40% by weight of atomic iodine and it is estimated that 3 mg of iodine is liberated daily per 100 mg of amiodarone ingested. Amiodarone is a potent inhibitor of 5-mono de-iodinase which converts T_4 to T_3 and also de-iodinates reverse T_3. This results in patients developing elevated TT_4, reduced TT_3 and elevated reverse T_3 levels while the serum TSH remains normal. Up to 10% of patients, however, develop overt thyroid dysfunction secondary to iodine overloading. This may consist of either hypo- or hyperthyroidism. There is some evidence that hyperthyroidism is commoner in areas with mild iodine deficiency, while hypothyroidism is commoner in areas where dietary iodine intake is high (Martino et al. 1984). Simple withdrawal of amiodarone does not usually resolve the disorder in that the drug accumulates in tissues and its principal metabolites have a half-life measured in months rather than hours (Holt et al. 1983).

Clinical Features

As in the case of hypothyroidism, thyrotoxicosis often has an atypical presentation in the elderly. Table 3.3 lists the prevalence of symptoms and signs found in patients with thyrotoxicosis over the age of 60 (Davis and Davis 1974). This shows that cardiovascular abnormalities with cachexia and weight loss are common. Few patients have excess sweating, increased appetite or diarrhoea, and although many have lid lag or retraction, frank exophthalmos is rare.

Many patients are anxious, nervous or hyperkinetic, but there is an important subgroup who are apathetic. This presentation described as apathetic thyrotoxicosis occurs characteristically in old age (Thomas et al. 1970). In addition to exhibiting mental symptoms described in Chap. 2, patients usually give a long history of ill health and have suffered profound weight loss. As in other old people with thyrotoxicosis, cardiovascular signs are prominent. Ankle swelling may also occur without other evidence of heart failure. Considerable concern has been expressed about the risk of arterial embolism in patients with atrial fibrillation and hyperthyroidism. Rates of embolism varying from 10% to 40% have been reported in different series (Forfar and Caldwell 1985).

Table 3.3. Prevalence of symptoms and signs in patients with thyrotoxicosis aged over 60 years (Davis and Davis 1974)

Symptoms	Percentage prevalence	Signs	Percentage prevalence
Tiredness	52	Cachexia	39
Excess sweating	9	Hyperkinetic	25
Weight loss	69	Apathetic	16
Palpitations	63	Warm moist skin	81
Angina	20	Lid lag	35
Breathlessness	66	Lid retraction	23
Increased appetite	11	Exophthalmos	8
Anorexia	36	Cardiomegaly	11
Diarrhoea	12	Bounding pulse	7
Constipation	26	Atrial fibrillation	39
Anxiety	60	Brisk tendon reflexes	26

The systematic complications of hyperthyroidism are discussed in more detail in Chap. 2.

Investigation

This is outlined in Chap. 12. It should be noted that elevation of both TT_4 and TT_3 is usual in hyperthyroidism, and that this applies also to the free hormones. The TT_3 is usually disproportionately elevated in relation to the TT_4 because of preferential secretion from the thyroid under a state of persistent stimulation. Indeed, some patients may have elevation solely of the TT_3. Such T_3 toxicosis is typical of patients with Graves' disease who relapse early on drug treatment and in patients with toxic adenomas. It is also a feature of mildly hyperthyroid individuals with a toxic multinodular goitre. Patients with T_3 toxicosis often go through a phase of sub-clinical hyperthyroidism (normal circulating thyroid hormone levels but a suppressed TSH and absent TSH response to TRH) and it has been claimed that up to 10% of patients with "lone" atrial fibrillation have this condition (Forfar et al. 1979).

The converse situation of true T_4 toxicosis is much less frequent and indeed its existence has been doubted. However, there is an increased ratio of T_4 to T_3 in patients with hyperthyroidism, due to iodine overload, thyroiditis or exogenous thyroxine administration. The ratio is particularly high if the condition is induced by amiodarone or if the hyperthyroidism is associated with a severe non-thyroidal illness inducing a low T_3 state. In these situations a suppressed TSH (by sensitive assay) or a "flat" TRH test may give additional information.

Management

The measures available for the management of hyperthyroidism include the use of beta-adrenoceptor antagonist drugs to relieve symptoms, the use of antithyroid drugs to block thyroid hormone synthesis and destruction of the thyroid gland using either ^{131}I or surgery.

Beta-adrenoceptor Antagonist Drugs

There is now extensive experience of the use of beta-blockers in the management of hyperthyroidism and propranolol has been used in this context for almost 20 years and has been intensively studied (Feely and Peden 1984). Unfortunately there is very little information about the effects of these drugs on elderly hyperthyroid patients as most of the reported studies have concentrated on younger patients. Thus there is little evidence on whether doses of these drugs need to be altered in old age.

The effects of propranolol and nadolol on reducing the heart rate are related to their plasma levels, and reduced renal and hepatic function may result in increased concentrations of both in old age (Feely and Stevenson 1978; Peden et al. 1982). There is wide inter-individual variation, however, so that dosage should be tailored to the needs of each patient (Feely and Peden 1984).

In hyperthyroidism beta-blockers reduce tachycardia, control atrial fibrillation and decrease tremor and anxiety. Propranolol, metoprolol, nadolol and sotalol have an additional mechanism of action in that they partially inhibit the conversion of T_4 to T_3, increasing the levels of reverse T_3.

Contra-indications to beta-blocker therapy in hyperthyroidism are the same as in euthyroid individuals. In elderly patients, beta-blockers have generally been reported as having a high incidence of adverse effects and they should be used with particular care in patients with heart failure.

Beta-blockers should be used in hyperthyroidism to effect the rapid relief of troublesome symptoms, particularly palpitation and tremor. They also are a useful adjunct to therapy while the effects of radio-iodine therapy are awaited. Propranolol is also indicated with digoxin for the control of atrial fibrillation in patients not in heart failure, as an adjunct to preparation for thyroid surgery, and in thyrotoxic crisis.

Antithyroid Drugs

The thioureylene group of drugs – carbimazole, its active metabolite methimazole and propylthiouracil (PTU) – have been widely used in the management of hyperthyroidism for over 40 years. They are concentrated in thyroid tissue, and inhibit thyroid hormone synthesis by complex effects on both the iodination of tyrosine residues and the coupling of iodo-tyrosines. They also suppress thyroid auto-antibody synthesis. Propylthiouracil has additional peripheral effects on the inhibition of conversion of T_4 to T_3.

These drugs are used as first-line therapy in many younger patients with hyperthyroidism, but in old age they are usually reserved for rendering patients euthyroid prior to destructive therapy. Their main function is to suppress hyperthyroidism while awaiting spontaneous remission of the condition. This is common in Graves' disease but unusual in toxic nodular goitre. A case can be made for long-term use of antithyroid drugs in a few elderly hyperthyroid patients shown to have low iodine uptake by tracer studies in whom ^{131}I may be ineffective, or in patients who do not wish definitive therapy by ^{131}I or surgery.

Carbimazole can be given once daily, the usual initial dose being 30–45 mg daily. Initial daily doses of PTU are generally ten times greater, and given three times daily because of the shorter half-life of the substance. The biochemical effect of these drugs precedes their clinical benefit and it takes 4–6 weeks to achieve a euthyroid state. At this stage the drug dose should be reduced by one-third and then titrated downwards to maintain euthyroidism. There is little information on whether ageing should modify the dose regimen.

The principal side-effects of antithyroid drugs are a rash and pruritis. These occur in up to 5% of patients, but cross-sensitivity between carbimazole and PTU is unusual. More worrying adverse effects relate to bone marrow suppression. These are dose-related and usually manifest as agranulocytosis which occurs suddenly during the first few weeks of treatment. The true incidence of this is unknown but is probably of the order of 1 in 500 patients. It is much more common in the older patients (Cooper et al. 1983).

The first symptom is usually sore throat or fever and patients should be instructed that if this happens they should discontinue treatment and contact their doctor immediately. If treated early, the condition is usually reversible.

Radio-iodine (^{131}I)

This is the treatment of choice for most elderly patients with hyperthyroid Graves' disease and for many with toxic nodular goitre. The dose is simple to administer and there is no long-term evidence of an increased risk of either thyroid cancer or other malignancies. There is no doubt that the treatment is effective, and the only contentious issues relate to dosage and to the use of adjunctive therapy with propranalol and antithyroid drugs while the patient becomes euthyroid.

The incidence of early hypothyroidism following ^{131}I has shown a progressive rise. This is true for the treatment of both Graves' disease and toxic nodular goitre and for both young and elderly patients (Holm et al. 1982). The reasons for the rising incidence are unclear but it has been suggested that an increased iodine content in the diet may play a part. In patients over the age of 70 with Graves' disease treatment with ^{131}I produces a rate of hypothyroidism 1 year afterwards of only 4% compared with one of 10% for patients aged 40 or younger. At 8 years of follow-up the respective rates were 35% and 46%. In patients with toxic nodular goitre the 1-year hypothyroidism rates for patients over 70 and 40 or less were 1% and 3% respectively while at 8 years the figures were 21% and 40% (Holm et al. 1982).

The apparent inevitability of hypothyroidism after ^{131}I therapy has prompted several authorities to suggest that patients should be given large "ablative" doses of ^{131}I in order to induce early permanent hypothyroidism as quickly as possible, so that lifelong thyroxine replacement therapy can then be established (Kendall-Taylor et al. 1984). This course was followed in patients up to 84 years of age, all of whom received initial doses of ^{131}I of 555 MBq (15 mCi). This may be particularly useful in atrial fibrillation where, in one study, 50% of patients given 600 MBq were hypothyroid by 6 months and many experienced reversion of atrial fibrillation to sinus rhythm (Scott et al. 1984).

Opinions vary on what constitutes a high dose of ^{131}I. Studies using average initial doses of ^{131}I of 245 MBq (Peden and Hart 1984) 555 MBq (Kendall-Taylor et al. 1984) and 600 MBq (Toft et al. 1981) have all achieved 50% hypothyroidism rates within 6 months. It should also be noted that even with large doses approximately 30% of patients are still euthyroid at three years.

In the face of a high incidence of hypothyroidism an alternative strategy has been the use of low doses of ^{131}I. In such regimens ^{131}I dosage is related to the estimated thyroid gland size expressed in terms of MBq/g thyroid tissue. This approach has the effect of causing hypothyroidism in only one-third of patients 10 years after treatment, but has the disadvantage that patients require a protracted period of control with antithyroid drugs before they become euthyroid.

In an elderly patient a good case can be made for early control of hyperthyroidism. In Graves' disease, initial doses of ^{131}I should be in the order of 370–555 mBq and with this approach many patients are hypothyroid by 6 months needing thyroxine replacement therapy. Once replacement thyroxine dosage has been stabilised the problem remains of long-term compliance in an elderly patient.

Various schemes have been advocated, including computer assisted follow-up registers.

Patients with toxic multinodular goitre tend to have lower ^{131}I uptakes than do patients with Graves' disease. These patients have, in the past, been given larger initial doses of [131]I (e.g. 555 MBq). The initial cure rate tends to be lower than for Graves' disease and hence further doses are often needed. The risk of hypothyroidism is lower.

If patients with a toxic adenoma (with suppression of the iodine uptake in the remainder of the gland) are to be treated with ^{131}I then larger doses should be used (e.g. 740 MBq initially). If iodine uptake in the rest of the gland is truly suppressed, then the rate of hypothyroidism should be low.

There is a risk of radiation thyroiditis in the early days (up to 2 weeks) after ^{131}I treatment. This may be accompanied by discharge of thyroid hormone into the circulation and exacerbation of hyperthyroidism even to the severity of a thyroid storm. This is a particular hazard in an elderly patient with cardiac disease. It can be avoided by pretreatment with antithyroid drugs. These should be discontinued a minimum of 48 h prior to dosing. If a patient has been particularly toxic, antithyroid drugs may be reinstituted 1 week after dosing, but if an "ablative" dose of ^{131}I has been given the antithyroid drugs can be discontinued after 6 weeks. An alternative is to treat the patient continuously with propranolol to prevent exacerbation of the hyperthyroid state after [131]I. This has the advantage that the biochemical status of the patient is more easily determined (Aro et al. 1981).

Surgery

In old age, surgery is usually reserved for patients with a large toxic multinodular goitre which may be causing local pressure effects. Such goitres often require large doses of ^{131}I to control hyperthyroidism and show little tendency to shrink with treatment so that pressure effects are not relieved. Debulking surgery usually controls hyperthyroidism (at least initially) and relieves pressure effects on the trachea.

Patients should normally be prepared for surgery with antithyroid drugs until euthyroid and be given Lugol's iodine pre-operatively. Preparation for surgery with beta-blockers with or without potassium iodine is much more convenient and rapid but this approach has not been systematically studied in elderly patients (Feely and Peden 1984).

Hemithyroidectomy is an effective treatment for toxic adenoma but in older patients ^{131}I is usually the preferred approach.

Treatment of Iodide-Induced Hyperthyroidism

This is usually mild and no treatment is required other than withdrawal of the iodide source. Propranolol may be helpful for short-term symptomatic control. Occasionally the hyperthyroidism is severe and treatment may be difficult. Propranolol is helpful in symptom control if an adequate dose is given. Antithyroid drugs block the further synthesis of thyroid hormones, but not the thyroid hormones already in store, so that control of the hyperthyroidism, even with large doses of antithyroid drugs, is likely to be slow. A low uptake of the isotope means that ^{131}I is ineffective. Surgery under full beta-adrenoceptor blockade may be undesirable in a patient who is elderly and who has a self-limiting condition.

Amiodarone-induced hyperthyroidism also presents major therapeutic difficulties (Himsworth 1985). Because of the long half-life of the drug, the patient has a large and long-lived iodine store. Beta-blockers may be contra-indicated because of the underlying cardiac problem but usually produce some symptomatic relief. Antithyroid drugs, as before, prevent synthesis of thyroid hormone but do not prevent the release of preformed hormone. Carbimazole should be used in an initial dose of 45 mg daily until the patient is euthyroid. Even after the euthyroid state is established, it should be maintained with this dose of carbimazole and with replacement triiodothyronine (T_3) therapy until all the tissue stores of amiodarone have been eliminated. This may take years. An alternative is to treat the patient with ^{131}I once iodine reserves have been sufficiently depleted to allow isotopic uptake by the thyroid (Himsworth 1985).

It has also been reported that patients with amiodarone induced hyperthyroidism may respond to prednisone in large doses of 50–100 mg daily. The rationale for this approach is unclear (Wimpfheimer et al. 1982).

Treatment of Thyroid Storm (Hyperthyroid Crisis)

This is a rare life-threatening condition characterised by a marked exacerbation of the hyperthyroid state with tachycardia, hyperpyrexia, agitation, confusion and heart failure or cardiovascular collapse. It is most commonly precipitated by infection or surgery in a patient with unsuspected hyperthyroidism or inadequately controlled by antithyroid drugs. It occasionally develops within 24 h of partial thyroidectomy and may be precipitated by thyroid hormone release following ^{131}I therapy.

Intravenous fluid and electrolyte support may be required along with appropriate sedation. Any associated infection should be vigorously treated. To prevent release of preformed thyroid hormone, iodine is given, either as Lugol's iodine (10 drops three times daily orally or via nasogastric tube), or as intravenous sodium iodide (1–2 g daily). Carbimazole, at least 60 mg daily, should be given orally via a nasogastric tube to block further synthesis of thyroid hormones. Intravenous hydrocortisone 100 mg six hourly is usually also given.

Propranolol has been particularly valuable in controlling the cardiovascular manifestations of a thyroid storm. This may be given orally as 80 mg initially and then six-hourly, or intravenously up to 5 mg (1 mg/min) six-hourly. When cardiac failure is present the patient should first be given digoxin and diuretics, and propranolol then administered cautiously.

Follow-up

In all forms of treatment for hyperthyroidism, follow-up is essential to assess efficacy and to identify hypothyroidism. After ^{131}I treatment for example, a review should be arranged at 6 weeks, 3 months, 6 months, 1 year and at annual intervals thereafter. Hypothyroidism 3 months after a dose of ^{131}I may be transient and approximately one-fifth of patients apparently hypothyroid at this time recover normal thyroid function. Such individuals often have no symptoms of hypothyroidism at this stage (Peden and Hart 1984). Since the clinical signs of hypothyroidism in old people are atypical, regular thyroid function tests at follow up are particularly important.

Goitre

Prevalence

Enlargement of the thyroid gland is four to five times as common in women as men (Tunbridge et al. 1977) (Fig. 3.2). There is a striking decline in its prevalence with increasing age so that it is half as common in women over 75 as those between 18 and 24, and does not occur at all in men over 75.

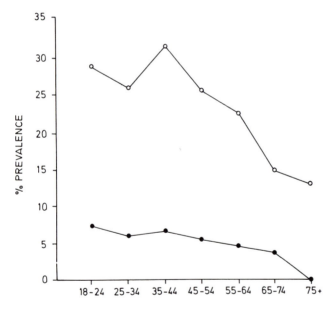

Fig. 3.2. Percentage prevalence of goitre related to age and sex (*solid circles*, men; *open circles*, women). (After Tunbridge et al. 1977.)

There have been no longitudinal studies of the condition, but it is likely that events including puberty, pregnancy, lactation and the menopause all have an effect on thyroid size. Thyroid size usually levels off or declines in youth or middle age, but there are instances where enlargement continues into old age.

Causes

In an elderly patient with a non-toxic goitre the following causes need to be considered: (1) multinodular goitre, (2) Hashimoto's thyroiditis, (3) carcinoma or lymphoma of the thyroid. Other causes are rare.

Clinical Features

In old age, goitres are often asymptomatic and are often identified coincidentally during the course of a physical examination. They feel firm and, since they are usually nodular, have a lumpy irregular surface.

Non-toxic goitre may present with local pressure effects such as dyspnoea, stridor (worse on reclining), dysphagia, venous obstruction, or an altered voice.

Haemorrhage into a cyst may cause sudden enlargement, pain and tenderness in a goitre. The discomfort usually settles within days and the swelling within weeks. A more serious problem is enlargement of the goitre down into the upper mediastinum with pressure on the trachea. Symptoms of tracheal obstruction may develop suddenly and the condition presents as a medical emergency (Warren 1979).

Differential Diagnosis

Hashimoto's Thyroiditis

In the earlier stages of this disease patients are usually euthyroid and occasionally thyrotoxic (How et al. 1981). Most ultimately become hypothyroid. It can be distinguished from multinodular goitre by the fact that it tends to present in a younger age group with diffuse firm enlargement of the thyroid. There are occasions, however, when the gland may feel nodular. The diagnosis can be confirmed by identifying high titres of thyroglobulin and thyroid microsomal antibodies or by needle biopsy.

Hyperthyroidism

This may be apparent clinically and should be confirmed by the appropriate tests of thyroid function.

Carcinoma

The clinical and investigational features of this are discussed in the next section. Various benign changes in a multinodular goitre may mimic malignancy. Haemorrhage into a cyst may produce sudden enlargement of the gland. Again, calcification of a cystic haemorrhage may produce a stony hard lump. Tracheal compression may result from both benign and malignant lesions, but laryngeal nerve damage is nearly always the result of the latter.

Investigation

Thyroid function tests progressing to TRH testing (if necessary) should be performed to confirm the thyroid status of the patient. Thyroid antibody studies are useful in confirming the suspected diagnosis of Hashimoto's disease. A thyroid isotope scan may show characteristic appearances in multinodular goitre or may show up a non-functioning area raising the suspicion of carcinoma. X-rays of the thoracic inlet may show calcification in a long-standing multinodular goitre and may also be useful for confirming evidence of tracheal compression. In doubtful cases, needle biopsy of the thyroid may be indicated. Ultrasound examination will confirm the presence of cysticareas.

Treatment

(1) *Multinodular Goitre.*   There is little point in using suppressive thyroxine therapy for this condition in elderly patients who in general terms are not particularly worried about cosmetic aspects. It is unlikely to be effective and if the gland is functioning autonomously there is the risk of inducing hyperthyroidism.

If the gland is causing significant mediastinal compression symptoms, surgery may be indicated. If the goitre has recurred after previous partial thyroidectomy, ^{131}I, at the largest possible out-patient dose, may shrink the gland. After surgery thyroxine should be given to prevent thyroid regrowth.

 If the gland is increasing in size rapidly and carcinoma is a possibility, then surgery is indicated.

If the gland is autonomous, i.e. the serum TSH is undetectable by sensitive assay or the TRH test is flat but with apparently normal free thyroid hormones, then regular observation for the development of overt hyperthyroidism is essential. Anecdotal reports suggest that in elderly patients with autonomously functioning multinodular goitres and atrial fibrillation treatment with ^{131}I may improve cardiac-function with reversion to sinus rhythm (Bruce et al. 1987) as has been reported in younger patients with so-called subclinical hyperthyroidism.

(2) *Hashimoto's Disease.*   If the goitre is not large and the patient euthyroid no treatment is indicated. If the size of the goitre is a problem or if there is elevation of TSH, suppressive thyroxine therapy may shrink the goitre. Clearly, if the patient is hypothyroid, thyroxine therapy is indicated.

(3) *Thyroid Cancer or Lymphoma.*   This is dealt with in a subsequent section.

Solitary Thyroid Nodules

The differential diagnosis of an apparently solitary thyroid nodule includes a multinodular goitre with a dominant nodule, a solitary toxic nodule or adenoma, a thyroid cyst, a benign adenoma (most commonly follicular), Hashimoto's disease and carcinoma or lymphoma of the thyroid. In general terms solitary thyroid nodules are more likely to be sinister (malignant) in younger than in older patients, in men than in women, if there is no family history of goitre and if the nodule is hard on palpation.

In the history, it is important to ask if there has been any history of irradiation to the neck and if there has been sudden enlargement with pain in the thyroid, suggesting haemorrhage into a cyst. Other relevant points to elicit are the rate of any thyroid enlargement and symptoms suggesting pressure on the trachea or oesophagus.

Examination should seek signs of hyperthyroidism or hypothyroidism, the latter suggesting the presence of Hashimoto's disease, anaplastic carcinoma or lymphoma. The thyroid should be carefully palpated as should the adjacent lymph nodes. The presence of enlarged lymph nodes suggests the presence of neoplasm although occasionally in Hashimoto's disease there may be local nodal enlargement.

Investigation includes biochemical confirmation of the thyroid status. The presence of thyroid auto-antibodies in high titres suggests the presence of Hashimoto's disease. Thyroid isotope scanning is often helpful in that if the nodule is a dominant one in a gland with other functioning and non-functioning areas, this suggests the presence of multinodular goitre. If there is a solitary functioning nodule with suppression of isotope intake elsewhere in the gland then this is likely to be a benign lesion. The size of the functioning nodule to some extent determines the risk of developing hyperthyroidism. If a nodule exceeds 3 cm in diameter, then this becomes particularly likely. About 10% of solitary poorly or non-functioning nodules are neoplastic. Ultrasound can be used to establish whether a lesion is cystic. Most cysts represent degeneration of solid nodules in which there often is a haemorrhagic component. Cyst aspiration is also useful and it is important that fluid be sent for cytological examination.

A further diagnostic approach in solid non-functioning or non-hyperfunctioning lesions is to perform a needle biopsy, using either fine needle aspiration cytology or a cutting-needle biopsy. The value of needle biopsies is dependent on local expertise in cytology and histopathology. Interpretation of a specimen is particularly difficult if the histology suggests that it is follicular in origin. In such lesions, evidence of venous or capillary invasion is very important. Unless there is substantial local expertise in the interpretation of needle biopsy specimens, it is best to proceed to surgical excision of the lesion for accurate diagnosis and prognosis.

Since the majority of solid thyroid nodules which show patchy uptake of isotope or non-function on isotope scanning are benign, the following approach is reasonable. If local pathological expertise is available, a needle biopsy should be taken. If the clinical features suggest malignancy, surgery for excision biopsy is indicated. If malignancy is unlikely an attempt to shrink the lesion with suppressive L-thyroxine treatment may be considered. If the lesion then shrinks in size, it is not malignant but if there is no shrinkage, the possibility of malignancy remains and the question of surgery for excision biopsy can again be addressed.

Thyroid Cancer

Prevalence

Malignant tumours of the thyroid gland are three times as common in women as in men (Christiansen et al. 1984). Its incidence rises from 2 per 100 000 aged 20–29, to 3.5 per 100 000 aged 60 to 69, reaching a peak of 7 per 100 000 aged 70–79. Table 3.4 shows the proportion of different types of thyroid malignancy (Staunton and Skeet, 1979). Patients with papillary, follicular and medullary tumours have mean ages between 40 and 60, while those with anaplastic carcinoma or lymphosarcoma are older with mean ages between 60 and 70 (Table 3.4). The finding of small occult thyroid cancers is particularly common in post mortem studies but the significance of such lesions is unclear (Harach et al. 1985).

Table 3.4. Proportion and mean ages of patients with different types of thyroid malignancy (Staunton and Skeet 1979)

Type	Percentage proportion	Mean age (years)
Papillary	31	45.6
Follicular	16	53.4
Medullary	3	52.1
Anaplastic	35	61.9
Lymphosarcoma	7	60.8
No histology	8	63.6

Pathology

Papillary and follicular carcinomas are tumours derived from cells lining the thyroid follicles. The former are characterised by tumour cells around a fibrovascular stalk. They are not encapsulated and infiltrate surrounding tissues. In the latter there are solid sheets of cells and though they are surrounded by a capsule, there is often invasion of both capsule and blood vessels. Follicular tumours may be capable of synthesising thyroxine and this has important diagnostic and therapeutic implications. Oxyphilic (Hürthle cell) varieties of differentiated thyroid cancer seem to be more prevalent in the elderly (Crile et al. 1985).

Medullary thyroid cancer is derived from the calcitonin secreting cells (C-cells) which lie between the follicles and are primarily tumours of younger patients who may have multiple endocrine adenomatosis.

Tumours made up of undifferentiated cells are highly invasive and there is often infiltration of surrounding structures including the trachea and recurrent laryngeal nerve.

Lymphomas of the thyroid often occur in older women with a history of chronic lymphocytic thyroiditis (Holm et al. 1985) or Hashimoto's disease (Hamburger et al. 1985). These tumours often show local invasion or involve neighbouring lymph nodes and are occasionally a manifestation of a generalised lymphoreticular malignancy.

Clinical Presentation

Patients usually consult a doctor because they feel a lump in their neck, or because invasion of surrounding structures causes symptoms such as choking or hoarseness (Christiansen et al. 1984). If the lesion is an anaplastic cancer, it is usually palpable as a mass, containing multiple hard nodules. It is often attached to surrounding tissues, the overlying skin may be cracked, and hard enlarged cervical lymph nodes are often palpable (Nel et al. 1985).

It is much less likely that an elderly patient will have a follicular or a papillary tumour. Since the former is usually encapsulated, it often presents as a single lump, not attached to surrounding tissues. Blood-borne metastases may cause a haemoptysis or a pathological fracture. A papillary tumour also usually presents as a hard discrete nodule but local lymph node enlargement is more common. Metastases of well differentiated follicular tumours are occasionally sufficiently functional to cause hyperthyroidism. Thyroid lymphoma usually presents as a firm non-tender mass and patients may be hypothyroid. There may be local lymph node enlargement (Burke et al. 1977; Hamburger et al. 1985).

Investigation

The initial investigation is to scan the neck following the intravenous injection of technetium-99m (Chap. 12). The tumour shows up as an area of low isotope uptake. An exception is a metabolically active follicular carcinoma in which there may be areas of isotope uptake in the thyroid and metastases. Conventional radiology can be useful in defining the extent of a lesion, or identifying pulmonary metastases. Isotopic scanning is the investigation of choice when searching for skeletal secondaries.

As mentioned in the previous section on the solitary thyroid nodule, needle biopsy of suspicious nodules is increasingly performed but is highly dependent on cytopathological and histopathological expertise. If this expertise is lacking, many clinicians would argue that the identification of low isotope uptake in a suspicious lesion provides suffcent justification for treating the lesion as malignant and proceeding to surgery with lobe resection for frozen section histology.

Prognosis

Table 3.5 shows the 5-year survival rates for different types of thyroid cancer and relates these to the age of the patients. The prognosis is appalling for anaplastic carcinoma at all ages and in all forms of thyroid cancer the prognosis is better for patients aged under 45 than patients 45 and over. A recent evaluation has suggested that the prognosis in follicular carcinoma is much worse in patients over the age of 60 years than in those under (Crile et al. 1985).

Table 3.5. Five-year survival for different types of thyroid cancer (Staunton and Skeet 1979)

Types of cancer	Percentage survival rate for age		
	0–44	45–59	60+
Papillary	97	62	54
Follicular	83	59	55
Anaplastic	33	7	14

Treatment

Anaplastic tumours should be treated with surgical resection, but total resection should only be attempted if there is no extracapsular extension (Wade 1983). In most instances treatment is limited to a central resection, followed by local radiotherapy. If this is ineffective, multiple cytotoxic therapy may be of temporary benefit. Overall, treatment has little influence on the appalling outcome of the condition.

The diagnosis of follicular carcinoma is usually made on the basis of histology from a lobectomy for a suspicious nodule (Wade 1983). The tumour is not usually multicentric. In old age it is rare for there to be no local or distant metastases, so that the initial operation is usually followed by local treatment with ^{131}I to ablate the thyroid remnant. L-Thyroxine is then given in a dose sufficient to suppress TSH secretion. This can then be discontinued periodically to permit whole body scanning with ^{131}I for detection of functional metastases. These, if detected, are treated with very large doses of ^{131}I.

In the elderly, most papillary carcinomas have invaded surrounding tissues by the time the diagnosis is established. Since the tumour may be multicentric, radical resection of the gland, sometimes with sacrifice of the recurrent laryngeal nerve, is indicated in all but the most frail (Wade 1983). Since the tumour is usually TSH-dependent, secretion of this should be suppressed with thyroxine in a dose sufficient to render the TSH undetectable without causing hyperthyroidism. In frail patients treatment with L-thyroxine without surgical resection may be appropriate.

In the presence of a well-differentiated thyroid cancer, the serum thyroglobulin level may be a useful tumour marker in detecting a recurrence. This is usually undetectable in patients free of metastatic disease receiving suppressive L-thyroxine. Lymphomas should be treated with external irradiation (Burke et al. 1977). The response depends upon the staging of the condition. If the lesion is confined to the thyroid, complete cure is possible in a large proportion of cases but once there is spread to local lymph nodes or beyond, the 5-year survival rate falls to 27% or less (Hamburger et al. 1985).

References

Aro A, Huttunen JK, Lamberg BA et al. (1981) Comparison of propanolol and carbimazole as adjuncts to iodine-131 therapy for hyperthyroidism. Acta Endocrinol (Copenh) 96: 321–327

Bahemuka M, Hodkinson HM (1975) Screening for hypothyroidism in elderly inpatients. Br Med J 2: 601–603

Bell GM, Todd WTA, Forfar JC et al. (1985) End-organ responses to thyroxine therapy in subclinical hypothyroidism. Clin Endocrinol 22: 83–89

Bruce SA, Rangedara DC, Lewis RR, Corless D (1987) Hyperthyroidism in elderly patients with atrial fibrillation and normal thyroid hormone measurements. J R Soc Med 80: 74–76

Burke JS, Butler JJ, Fuller LM (1977) Malignant lymphomas of the thyroid. A clinical pathologic study of 35 patients including ultrastructural observations. Cancer 39: 1587–1602

Caplan RH, Wickus G, Glasser JE et al. (1981) Serum concentrations of iodothyronines in elderly subjects: decreased triiodothyronine (T3) and free T_3 index. J Am Geriatr Soc 29: 19–24

Chopra IJ, Huang TS, Beredo A (1985) Evidence for an inhibitor of extrathyroidal conversion of T_4 to $3,5,3'$ T_3 in sera of patients with non-thyroidal illnesses. J Clin Endocrinol Metab 60: 666–672

Chopra IJ, Teco GNG, Mead JF et al. (1985) Relationships between serum free fatty acids and thyroid hormone binding inhibitors in non-thyroidal illnesses. J Clin Endocrinol Metab 60: 980–984

Christiansen SB, Sjungberg O, Tibblin S (1984) Thyroid carcinoma in Malmö, 1960–1977. Epidemiologic, clinical and prognostic findings in a defined urban population. Cancer 53: 1625–1633

Cooper DS, Goldmin D, Levin AA et al. (1983) Agranulocytosis associated with antithyroid drugs. Ann Intern Med 98: 26–29

Crile G, Portius I, Hawk WA (1985) Survival of patients with follicular carcinoma of the thyroid gland. Surg Gynecol Obstet 160: 409–413

Cropper CFJ (1973) Hypothyroidism in psychiatric patients – ankle jerk reaction time as a screening technique. Gerontol Clin 15: 15–24

Davis PJ, Davis FB (1974) Hyperthyroidism in patients over the age of 60 years. Clinical features in 85 patients. Medicine 53: 161–181

Doniach D, Bottazzo GF, Russell RCG (1979) Goitrous auto-immune thyroiditis (Hashimoto's disease). Clin Endocrinol Metab 8: 63–80

Evered D, Young ET, Ormston BJ, Menzies R, Smith PA, Hall R (1973) Treatment of hypothyroidism. A reappraisal of thyroxine therapy. Br Med J 3: 131–134

Falkenberg M, Kagedal B, Norr A (1983) Screening of an elderly female population for hypo- and hyperthyroidism by use of a thyroid hormone panel. Acta Med Scand 214: 361–365

Feely J, Peden NR (1984) Use of β-adrenoceptor blocking drugs in hyperthyroidism. Drugs 27: 425–446

Feely J, Stevenson IH (1978) The effect of age and hyperthyroidism on plasma propranolol steady state concentration. Br J Clin Pharmacol 6: 446P

Forfar JC, Caldwell GC (1985) Hyperthyroid heart disease. Clin Endocrinol 14: 491–508

Forfar JC, Miller HC, Toft AD (1979) Occult thyrotoxicosis: a treatable cause of "idiopathic" atrial fibrillation. Am J Cardiol 44: 9–12

Forrester CF (1963) Coma in myxoedema. Arch Intern Med 111: 700–743

Fraser WD, Biggart EM, O'Reilly DSJ, Gray HW, McKillop JH, Thomson JA (1986) Are biochemical tests of thyroid function of any value in monitoring patients receiving thyroxine replacement. Br Med J 293: 808–810

Greenwood RM, Daly JG, Himsworth RC (1985) Hyperthyroidism and the impalpable thyroid. Clin Endocrinol 22: 583–587

Hall R, Anderson J, Smart GA, Besser M (1980) Fundamentals of clinical endocrinology. 3rd ed. Pitman Medical, Tunbridge Wells 165

Hamburger JI, Miller JM, Kim SR (1985) Lymphoma of the thyroid. Ann Intern Med 99: 685–693

Harach HR, Franssila KD, Wasenius VM (1985) Occult papillary carcinoma of the thyroid. A "normal" finding in Finland. A systematic autopsy study. Cancer 56: 531–538

Himsworth RL (1985) Hyperthyroidism with a low iodine uptake. Clin Endocrinol Metab 14: 397–416

Hodkinson HM, Denham MJ (1977) Thyroid function in the elderly in the community. Age Ageing 6: 67–70

Holm LE (1982) Changing annual incidence of hypothyroidism after Iodine-131 Therapy for hyper-
     thyroidism. J Nucl Med 23: 108–112
Holm LE, Lundell G, Israelsson A, Dahlqvist I (1982) Incidence of hypothyroidism occurring long
     after Iodine-131 therapy for hyperthyroidism. J Nucl Med 23: 103–107
Holm LE, Blomgren H, Löwhagen T (1985) Cancer risks in patients with chronic lymphocytic
     thyroiditis. N Engl J Med 312: 601–604
Holt DW, Incker GT, Jackson PR, Storey GC (1983) Amiodarone pharmacokinetics. Am Heart J
     106: 840–847
How J, Topliss D, Lewis M et al (1981) Clearing up confusion about goitre. Geriatrics 36: 111–118
Hurley JY (1983) Thyroid disease in the elderly. Med Clin N Am 67: 497–516
Hylander B, Rosenqvist V (1985) Treatment of myxoedema coma – factors associated with fatal out-
     come. Acta Endocrinol (Copenh) 108: 65–71
Jeffreys PM (1972) The prevalence of thyroid disease in patients admitted to a geriatric department.
     Age Ageing 1: 33–40
Kendall-Taylor P, Keir MJ, Ross WM (1984) Ablative radio-iodine therapy for hyperthyroidism: long
     term follow up study. Br Med J 289: 361–363
Leger AF, Massin JP, Laurent MF et al. (1984) Iodine induced thyrotoxicosis: An analysis of eighty
     five consecutive cases. Eur J Clin Invest 14: 449–455
Levy RP, Jensen JB, Lewis VG et al. (1981) Serum thyroid hormone abnormalities in psychiatric dis-
     ease. Metabolism 30: 1060–1064
MacLellan WJ (1985) Hypothermia. In: Lye M (ed) Acute geriatric medicine. MTP Press, pp 75–92
Mardell RJ, Gamlen TR, Winton MRJ (1985) High sensitivity assay of thyroid stimulating hormone
     in patients receiving thyroxine for primary hypothyroidism and thyroid cancer. Br Med J 290:
     355–356
Martino E, Safran M, Aghini-Lombardi F et al. (1984) Environmental iodine uptake and thyroid dys-
     function during chronic amiodarone therapy. Ann Intern Med 101: 28–34
McPherson JN, Isles TE, Peden NR, Crooks J (1982) Importance of thyroxine in suppressing secretion
     of thyroid stimulating hormone. Br Med J 284: 1479
Nel CJC, Van Heerden JA, Goellner JR et al. (1985) Anaplastic carcinoma of thyroid: a
     clinicopathologic study of 82 cases. Mayo Clin Proc 60: 51–58
Nofal MM, Bierwaltes WH, Patno ME (1966) Treatment of hyperthyroidism with sodium iodide
     I-131, JAMA 197: 605–610
Pearce CJ, Himsworth RL (1982) Thyrotoxicosis factitia. N Engl J Med 307: 1708–1709
Peden NR, Hart IR (1984) The early development of transient and permanent hypothyroidism follow-
     ing radioiodine therapy for hyperthyroid Graves' disease. Can Med Assoc J 130: 1141–1144
Peden NR, Isles TE, Stevenson IH, Crooks J (1982) Nadolol in thyrotoxicosis. Br J Clin Pharmacol
     13: 835–840
Rendell M, Salmon D (1985) "Chemical Hyperthyroidism". The significance of elevated serum
     thyroxine levels in L-thyroxine treated individuals. Clin Endocrinol 22: 693–700
Ridgeway EC, Cooper DS, Walker H, Rodbard D, Maloof F (1981) Peripheral responses to thyroid
     hormone before and after L-thyroxine therapy in patients with subclinical hypothyroidism. J Clin
     Endocrinol Metab 53: 1238–1262
Rosenbaum RL, Bazel US (1982) Levothyroxine replacement dose for primary hypothyroidism
     decreases with age. Ann Intern Med 96: 53–55
Sawin CT, Chopra D, Azizi F et al. (1979) The ageing thyroid – increased prevalence of elevated serum
     thyrotrophin levels in the elderly. JAMA 242: 247–250
Sawin C, Herman T, Molitch ME et al. (1983) Ageing and the thyroid. Decreased requirement for
     thyroid hormone in older hypothyroid patients. Am J Med 75: 206–209
Scott GR, Forfar JC, Toft AD (1984) Graves' disease and atrial fibrillation: the case for even higher
     doses of therapeutic Iodine-131. Br Med J 289: 399–400
Staunton MD, Skeet RG (1979) Thyroid cancer: prognosis in 469 patients. Br J Surg 66: 643–647
Stewart JC, Vidor GI (1976) Thyrotoxicosis induced by iodine contamination of food – a common
     unrecognised condition. Br Med J 1: 372–375
Studer H, Peter HJ, Gerber H (1985) Toxic nodular goitre. Clin Endocrinol Metab 14: 351–372
Thomas FB, Mazzaferri EL, Skillman TG (1970) Apathetic thyrotoxicosis: a distinctive clinical and
     laboratory entity. Ann Intern Med 72: 679–685
Toft A, Campbell I, Seth J (1981) Diagnosis and management of endocrine diseases. Oxford,
     Blackwell Scientific Publications, p 214

Tunbridge WMG, Evered DC, Hall R et al. (1977) The spectrum of thyroid disease in a community: The Whickam Survey. Clin Endocrinol 7: 481–493

Vagenakis AG, Wang C, Burger A et al. (1972) Iodide induced thyrotoxicosis in Boston. N Engl J Med 287: 523–527

Wade JS (1983) The management of malignant thyroid tumours. Br J Surg 70: 253–255

Warren CPW (1979) Acute respiratory failure and tracheal obstruction in the elderly with benign goitres. Can Med Assoc J 121: 191–194

Wenzel KW (1981) Pharmacological interference with in vitro tests of thyroid function. Metabolism 30: 717–732

Wimpfheimer C, Staubli M, Schadelin J, Studer J, Studer H (1982) Prednisone in amiodarone induced thyrotoxicosis. Br Med J 284: 1835–1836

4 Diabetes Mellitus: Clinical Aspects

Diabetes mellitus is one of the most important causes of morbidity and mortality in old age. Since impaired carbohydrate tolerance appears to be a normal feature of ageing, there has been a prolonged debate as to whether non-insulin-dependent diabetes in the elderly is an ageing phenomenon or a disease process. Again, many of the atherosclerotic complications of diabetes mellitus closely resemble those of normal ageing, so that the question has been raised as to whether or not the disorder causes an exacerbation of the ageing process (Kent 1976). Far from being of mere academic interest, these issues are of fundamental importance in the diagnosis and management of diabetes mellitus and its complications in the elderly.

Diagnosis

Both mean fasting and post-prandial blood glucose concentrations rise with increasing age, so that in old age some elevation in these could be considered as being "normal". One approach to this would be to construct a nomogram which related blood glucose concentrations to age (Andres 1971). The alternative view is that no matter the age of the patient, persistent elevation of the blood glucose concentration above the normal for young adults is potentially harmful (Williams 1981).

Whatever the argument, from a practical point of view, an elderly patient with typical symptoms of diabetes mellitus with a random venous plasma glucose of > 11.1 mmol/l, or a fasting one of > 7.8 mmol/l, should be considered to have the condition (Keen and Ng Tang Fui 1982). These are the levels above which the characteristic microvascular complications of diabetes occur. Patients with random and fasting plasma glucose levels of less than 7.8 mmol/l should be labelled as not having the condition. It should be noted that venous whole blood glucose concentrations are approximately 1.0 mmol/l lower than equivalent plasma values.

Where glucose levels lie between the two sets of values a glucose tolerance test should be performed. A 75 g dose of oral glucose is given, and a specimen withdrawn to measure the plasma glucose 1 h and 2 h later. If the value is > 11.1 mmol/l, and the patient has symptoms, then diabetes mellitus is diagnosed. In asymptomatic patients the diagnosis should only be made if glucose levels at both 1 and 2 h are >11.1 mmol/l. Patients with a fasting plasma glucose < 7.8 mmol/l and 2-h values between 7.8 and 11.1 mmol/l, are considered to have impaired glucose tolerance (IGT), sometimes known in North America as hyperglycaemia of ageing. Approximately 2% per annum of individuals with IGT will go on to develop overt diabetes mellitus, while a proportion revert to having normal glucose tolerance (Keen and Ng Tang Fui 1982).

In the past, urine samples have been tested for glucose, as a screening test for diabetes; but the amount of glucose in the urine is a very poor guide to the blood glucose level in any age group, and poses particular problems in old age where the renal threshold for the excretion of glucose is often grossly elevated (Hayford et al. 1983).

In addition to diagnosing the condition, it is necessary to consider whether diabetes mellitus is insulin-dependent (IDDM) or non-insulin-dependent (NIDDM). In one study, 40 (10%) of 398 newly diagnosed diabetics aged 65 or over were initially identified as requiring insulin; 16 of these died within 2 years, suggesting that in the elderly, insulin dependency is of grave prognostic significance. Only eight of the remainder continued on insulin, and it was probable that only three of these were truly insulin-dependent. This suggests that in a clinic population of newly diagnosed elderly diabetics, only around 3% have true insulin dependence (Kilvert et al. 1984).

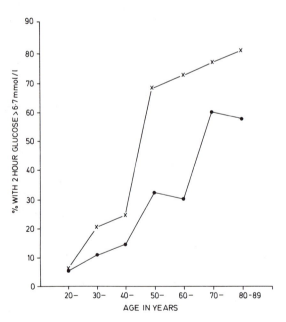

Fig. 4.1. Proportion of men (*circles*) and women (*crosses*) with abnormal glucose tolerance test in Bedford survey. (After Butterfield 1964.)

Prevalence

There is a striking increase in the prevalence of diabetes mellitus with increasing age (Butterfield 1964). In the Bedford study of the population in general, 57% of men and 86% of women over 80 had an abnormal glucose tolerance test (Fig. 4.1). Even if the large proportion with marginal abnormalities were excluded, there remained around a quarter of men and rather more than half of women over 80 with a blood glucose concentration in excess of 11.1 mmol/l 2 h after a 50 g oral dose of glucose. Data from the Framingham study suggests that the prevalence of glucose intolerance and diabetes mellitus is rising, and there are independent associations for these disorders with both increasing age and increasing body weight (Wilson et al. 1986). A community-based study in Poole, England, of all known diabetics in a well-defined population revealed that over half (52.2%), were of age 65 years or over with a 3.1% prevalence in those over 65 (Petri et al. 1986). The prevalence increased with age to 45.7 per 1000 in men and 29 per 1000 in women aged 75 or over.

Aetiology and Pathogenesis

The vast majority of elderly diabetics are obese and non-insulin-dependent. The pathogenesis of their diabetes remains controversial. In the obese it appears that diabetes is preceded by a period of hyperinsulinaemia and peripheral insulin resistance. As these patients become overtly hyperglycaemic there is a reduction of insulin secretion, which is particularly marked in the first 3 min after an intravenous hyperglycaemic stimulus (first phase), but also occurs in the second prolonged phase of insulin secretion (Ward et al. 1986). The loss of insulin secretion exacerbates the hyperglycaemia. Obese patients with mild impairment of glucose tolerance are also insulin resistant, a result of reduced insulin binding at peripheral sites.

In frank non-insulin-dependent diabetes in both obese and non-obese patients with fasting hyperglycaemia, there is severe insulin resistance with excessive rates of hepatic glucose production. There are also abnormalities, both of insulin binding and of insulin action on various enzyme systems within cells after insulin binding (post-receptor defect) (Kolterman 1987). What remains unclear and controversial is what comes first – is it insulin resistance, which eventually results in hyperglycaemia and reduced insulin secretion or is it defective insulin secretion? To complicate matters further, however, there is also evidence that hyperglycaemia inhibits insulin secretion and that this inhibition may be reversed by restoring normoglycaemia. It was recently shown that non-diabetic relatives of patients with NIDDM (i.e. high risk individuals) had a more marked reduction in insulin secretion than an increase in insulin resistance, suggesting that defective islet beta-cell function was the primary defect in NIDDM (O'Rahilly et al. 1986). What is clear is that, once developed, NIDDM is characterised by both decreased insulin secretion and sensitivity.

Genetic Factors

A study on twins and first-degree relatives of subjects with non-insulin-dependent diabetes demonstrated that genetic factors are extremely important in the development of this condition, with concordance between identical twins verging on 100% (Pyke 1979). However, epidemiological reviews of the same races in "primitive" and "developed" cultures have produced convincing evidence that environmental factors play a critical part in the constitutional tendency to NIDDM declaring itself (Zimmet 1982). Although there are underlying genetic factors in diabetes mellitus it is important that environmental factors receive appropriate emphasis, since only these can be influenced by treatment and changes in lifestyle.

Obesity

Obese subjects are insulin-resistant, and have adipocytes and skeletal muscle cells which show a reduced insulin-induced glucose uptake (Jung, 1984). The type of obesity and body fat distribution is important in this context and it is clear that individuals with a central distribution of body fat (android) have an increased prevalence of diabetes, in comparison to those individuals with an excessive deposition of fat on hips and thighs (gynaecoid). This being the case, the ratios of hip and waist measurements are useful in predicting the risk of diabetes (Ohlson et al. 1985). In the Framingham study, the body mass index was an important independent predictor for development of diabetes during follow-up, in both men and women (Wilson et al. 1986), so that increasing age and increasing relative weight may both be important in the development of diabetes mellitus. The role that the increasing relative proportion of adipose to muscle tissue with ageing, plays in the development of glucose tolerance in the elderly is unclear. However, there is the circumstantial evidence that muscle accounts for 83% of the uptake of an infused glucose load compared with only 1% of the relatively inactive adipose tissue (De Fronzo and Ferrannini 1987). Therefore, a change in the ratio might be expected to increase insulin resistance.

Physical Activity

NIDDM is more common in sedentary workers than in those of comparable weights engaged in moderate or heavy physical activity (Zimmet 1982). The converse is that a programme of physical activity is effective in increasing glucose utilisation in both normal and diabetic subjects (Vranic and Berger 1979). It is therefore possible that the decline in physical activity often associated with ageing and disability may be a significant factor in the high prevalence of NIDDM in old age.

Diet

It is uncertain whether the quality as well as the quantity of carbohydrate in the diet has an effect on glucose metabolism (Zimmet 1982). Suggestions that a high intake of refined sugar, or a reduced intake of fibre, exacerbate the tendency to NIDDM have not gained general acceptance.

Exocrine Pancreatic Disease

Diabetes mellitus may be the presenting feature of exocrine pancreatic disease, though chronic pancreatitis is usually characterised by pain. There is an excess of pancreatic cancer among patients with diabetes mellitus. It appears that this excess occurs among elderly patients developing diabetes late in life, rather than those in whom diabetes is long-standing. Carcinoma of the pancreas should be considered, therefore, when an elderly diabetic continues to lose weight, despite treatment or if his diabetes proves difficult to control (Morris and Nabarro 1984).

Drug Treatment

Several drugs widely used in old people impair carbohydrate metabolism, and may precipitate or exacerbate diabetes mellitus. The problem is discussed in more detail in Chap. 11.

Clinical Presentation and Complications

There is a wide spectrum of clinical presentation of diabetes mellitus in the elderly. Many apparently asymptomatic patients are identified by the presence of glycosuria or an elevated blood glucose during evaluation of many of the disorders which may or may not be related to the diabetes. A few have mild or moderate symptoms referrable to diabetes mellitus, particularly polydipsia and polyuria.

An infection is a common presenting feature in women and candidal vulvovaginitis often is the first indication of diabetes. Patients occasionally present with more severe symptoms, such as marked polydipsia, polyuria, weight loss and ketonuria. Keto-acidosis may be precipitated by an infection or other intercurrent stress, such as myocardial infarction. More commonly, however, severe metabolic decompensation in the elderly patient manifests itself as a hyperglycaemic hyperosmolar non-ketotic state.

Hypertension

It is becoming increasingly clear that there is a ubiquitous relationship between NIDDM and hypertension. In a large Israeli study, there was an association between glucose intolerance, and hypertension unrelated to age or degree of obesity, and plasma insulin levels had a positive relationship to blood pressure (Modan et al. 1985). In the Framingham study, at all ages patients with diabetes had 2 to

2.5 times the prevalence of raised systolic blood pressure as non-diabetics (Wilson et al. 1986). Again, this was unrelated to the degree of obesity. Investigations at Whitehall demonstrated that, at baseline and 2 h, blood glucose levels were related to systolic and diastolic blood pressure, again irrespective of age and degree of obesity (Jarrett 1985).

Though the relationship between hypertension and diabetes may be of great importance in the pathogenesis of the complications of diabetes, this should be differentiated from the situation in long-standing diabetes where a nephropathy gives rise to a secondary hypertension. Most hypertensive patients with NIDDM do not have overt nephropathy.

Atherosclerotic Vascular Disease

Atherosclerotic vascular disease (ASVD), presenting as coronary heart disease (CHD), cerebrovascular disease, peripheral vascular disease (PVD), or a combination of these is responsible for much of the increased morbidity and mortality in elderly patients with diabetes mellitus. CHD and PVD are particularly common in women with diabetes when the normal protection of women from vascular disease is lost.

Hyperglycaemia itself is an important risk factor for ASVD, and, in the Whitehall study, individuals in the top 5% of the glucose tolerance distribution were at particular risk from coronary or cerebrovascular episodes (Jarrett 1985). This relationship has also been found in other populations and other forms of ASVD (Pyorala et al. 1987). In the middle-aged and elderly, the increased risk is present at the time of diagnosis, and usually unrelated to the known duration of the diabetes, suggesting that prolonged asymptomatic diabetes or impaired glucose tolerance (i.e. relative hyperglycaemia) may be important risk factors.

There is also evidence that hyperinsulinaemia may increase the risk of ASVD (Pyorala et al. 1987). As stated earlier, hypertension in patients with NIDDM is also a major risk factor for the development of ASVD. It may also be that cigarette smoking interacts with hyperglycaemia as a cause of cardiovascular disease in elderly diabetics (Suarez et al. 1984).

Plasma lipid and lipoprotein abnormalities are particularly common in patients with NIDDM, with plasma total and very low density lipoprotein cholestrol (VLDL) levels being elevated and high density lipoprotein cholesterol (CHDL) decreased. These may result from abnormalities of lipoprotein metabolism with increased hepatic production and decreased clearance of lipoprotein due to decreased activity of insulin-dependent lipoprotein lipase. The clearance of low density lipoprotein (LDL) in diabetes may also be altered by non-enzymatic glycosylation (Pyorala et al. 1987).

There is also evidence that diabetes alters haemostasis by changes in the vascular endothelium, platelets, blood clotting and fibrolysis, shifting their complex relationship in a more thrombogenic direction (Pyorala et al. 1987).

Cerebrovascular Disease

It has been observed that over a 16-year period, middle-aged and elderly diabetic patients are two-and-a-half times as likely to sustain, and three-and-a-half times as likely to die from a stroke as non-diabetic contemporaries, the risk being even higher in women (Garcia et al. 1974).

As with non-diabetics, occlusive carotid artery disease is associated with the presence of coronary artery disease and in a group of 191 diabetics undergoing carotid surgery there was double the rate of death from myocardial infarction compared with non-diabetics (Campbell et al. 1984). In making the diagnosis of diabetes in the immediate post-stroke period it is important to recognise that the stress of the stroke itself may cause a temporary hyperglycaemia.

Coronary Artery Disease

Men and women over 60 with diabetes are two to two-and-a-half times as likely to have ischaemic heart disease as their non-diabetic contemporaries (Jarrett 1985). It is important, therefore, to screen for diabetes in patients with angina or myocardial infarction. There is the proviso that, as with stroke, there may be a temporary and stress-related elevation of the blood glucose concentration after myocardial infarction.

Peripheral Vascular Disease

There is an extremely high incidence of peripheral vascular disease (PVD) in men and women with NIDDM (Kreines et al. 1985) (Fig. 4.2). In the Framingham study of diabetic patients aged 70–79, approximately 10% had PVD, with 40%

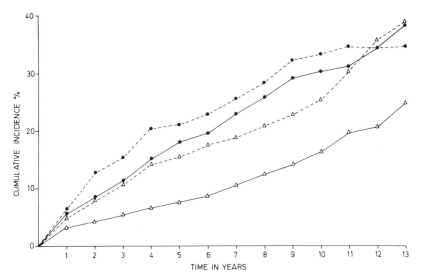

Fig. 4.2. Cumulative incidence of intermittent claudication (IC) and a non-palpable dorsalis pedis pulse (NPDPP) in men (*circles*) and women (*triangles*) with NIDDM (*broken lines*; controls shown by *solid lines*). (After Kreines et al. 1985.)

having some evidence of ASVD (Wilson et al. 1986). NIDDM increases the risk of a lower-limb amputation with over half of all non-traumatic amputations being carried out in elderly diabetic patients (Tattersall 1984). The pattern of PVD in elderly diabetics is different to that of non-diabetics, PVD in elderly diabetics having a particular predeliction for vessels below rather than above the knee (Edmonds 1986).

Small Vessel Disease

Diabetes also produces changes in small blood vessels. The most important of these is thickening of the capillary basement membrane (Vracko 1982). These changes are of particular relevance in the renal glomeruli and in the retina but may also accentuate the effects of large artery disease in the heart, limbs and nerves.

Examples are that small blood vessel changes in the heart may result in a diabetic cardiomyopathy with congestive heart failure, while those in the skin may exacerbate ulceration in a tissue already compromised by atherosclerosis and peripheral nerve degeneration, and occlusion of capillaries in peripheral nerves correlates with the severity of a neuropathy (Dyck et al. 1985).

Mental Function

Autopsies on patients with diabetes mellitus have identified far more extensive cerebral atherosclerosis, and small vessel damage than in controls (Wilkinson 1981). One manifestation of this was that patients with NIDDM (age 55–74) had greater evidence of defective memory retrieval when compared with non-diabetic controls (Perlmuter et al. 1984).

A far more common problem is that of an acute confusional state associated with hypoglycaemia. This is more common in patients treated with insulin, but can also occur during treatment with sulphonylureas, particularly if these have a long duration of action and cause cumulation. A diagnostic difficulty in old people is that autonomic degeneration may mask secondary features of hypoglycaemia such as anxiety, tremor, pallor, sweating and tachycardia. Single or repeated attacks of hypoglycaemic coma may give rise to permanent changes in the cerebral cortex (Brierley 1976). Gross changes consist of enlargement of cerebral ventricles, and cortical atrophy with particular shrinkage of the hippocampi. Histological examination reveals a laminar neuronal degeneration with particular involvement of the third and fifth cortical cellular layers. There may also be diffuse demyelination and gliosis in the white matter. These changes have usually been identified in patients with massive overdoses of insulin and it is less clear whether minor but recurrent attacks of hypoglycaemia lead to similar changes.

Peripheral Neuropathy

One of the most insidious but serious complications of NIDDM is peripheral nerve degeneration in the lower extremities (Ward 1982). There is good epidemiological evidence that this is a direct consequence of poor metabolic control of diabetes. A variety of pathological features have been described, including segmental demyelination, axonal degeneration, and Schwann cell damage, but it may be that these are secondary to obstructive changes in the vasa nervorum.

There is also evidence that other metabolic abnormalities are important, particularly increased activity of the polyol pathway, with accumulation of polyols, principally sorbitol. This causes a reduction of intracellular myoinositol which in turn results in an abnormal initiation of membrane phosphoinositides, which may be important in the pathogenesis of diabetic neuropathy (Greene 1986).

A number of patterns of diabetic neuropathy are recognised. Mononeuropathies commonly affect the cranial nerves particularly III, IV and VI, but may affect peripheral nerves (e.g. the peroneal nerve causing foot drop). Such a mononeuropathy may indeed be the presenting clinical feature of diabetes mellitus. The lesion usually develops suddenly with resolution of over 6–12 weeks. Proximal motor neuropathy (diabetic amyotrophy) typically causes asymmetric pain and weakness in the thighs associated with a loss of knee reflexes. The common polyneuropathies are acute sensory polyneuropathy usually involving the feet and causing unpleasant paraesthesiae, and chronic sensorimotor neuropathy causing loss of sensation with wasting of the small muscles of the feet. When loss of sensation is the only feature it may be difficult to distinguish changes due to diabetes from those of normal ageing. The trunk may also be affected by diabetic neuropathy with symptoms usually in a radicular distribution causing chest or abdominal pain.

Careful clinical evaluation and physiological blood-flow studies may be required to distinguish the effects of nerve degeneration from those of peripheral vascular disease. Electrophysiological studies usually are of limited value in old people in that they fail to distinguish peripheral changes due to diabetes from those of ageing. They are occasionally of more value in situations such as proximal motor neuropathy.

A more serious consequence is that of ulceration and infection of the neuropathic diabetic foot resulting from reduced pain sensation. The lesion often starts as a small traumatic painless cut or blister, but expands to form an extensive area of infection, necrosis and ulceration. A poor peripheral circulation, a reduced immunological response to infection, and the fact that an old person with poor eyesight and osteoarthritis may not see the lesion, all exacerbate the problem. Ultimately, the foot becomes gangrenous, resulting in immobilisation, surgery, amputation, septicaemia or death.

Autonomic Neuropathy

Diabetes sometimes causes degeneration of both the sympathetic and parasympathetic nervous systems. Important clinical consequences of this are postural hypotension, bladder dysfunction, impotence, an increased risk of hypothermia and gut disturbances, particularly diarrhoea. A variety of tests have been devised to identify autonomic degeneration (Ewing and Clarke 1982). These are relatively simple, but problems of cooperation with testing, and the overlap between the effects of ageing and those of diabetes mean that they are of little value in the routine evaluation of elderly patients (MacLennan, personal observation).

Vision

Diabetes mellitus causes the premature formation of a lens cataract with an appearance indistinguishable from that found in non-diabetic subjects in old age (Karasik et al. 1984). Most studies suggest that the increased prevalence of cataracts in diabetes is confined to women. Further, although the overall prevalence of cataracts in diabetics increases with age, the relative difference in the risk of cataracts between diabetic and non-diabetic patients is greater under the age of 40. Even over the age of 60, however, women with diabetes are at least four times as likely to have cataracts as others. Other factors increasing the risk of cataracts are the duration of the diabetes, and poor control of blood glucose levels.

Mechanisms responsible for this excess of senile cataract among diabetics include activation of the polyol pathway, which results in a decrease in the concentration of reduced glutathione, a substance important in preventing the glycosylation and carbamylation of lens proteins. In this situation they are more susceptible to cross-linking, resulting in a loss of lens opacity (Bron and Cheng 1986).

Retinopathy

Diabetic retinopathy is more common in old people but this is related to the fact that more of them have had diabetes for longer (Segal et al. 1984). Age has no independent effect on the incidence of the condition in older patients. Unlike cataract, retinopathy is equally common in men and women. The quality of control of blood glucose levels has an important influence on the incidence and progression of the condition. About one in ten patients with diabetes over the age of 60 have retinopathy at the time of diagnosis and 5 years after this the proportion has risen to one-third. Patients developing retinopathy are likely to have higher blood glucose levels than those not. Blood pressure also has an adverse effect on the progression of retinopathy.

The pattern of retinopathy differs between young patients with IDDM and older patients with NIDDM. The latter often suffer from a maculopathy – scattered or circular (circinate) groups of hard exudates involving the macular part of the retina. Circinate groups of hard exudates are often associated with macular oedema. This may not be apparent on monocular ophthalmoscopy and often requires binocular stereoscopic equipment for detection.

The presence of macular oedema is sinister, as it spreads to cause loss of central vision. This can be identified in the diabetic clinic by looking for a decline in central visual acuity. The presence of maculopathy does not preclude progression of a retinopathy to preproliferative and proliferative forms typical of young patients with IDDM.

Given the high prevalence of retinopathy in elderly patients and the concomitant high prevalence of cataract, it is important that in diabetic patients with cataract a formal ophthalmological opinion is obtained, so that these conditions can be adequately assessed and treated if necessary.

Renal Disease

Microvascular changes in the limbs and retina are reflected by similar abnormalities in the kidneys of diabetics, giving rise to the problems of proteinuria and renal impairment. Pathological changes in the glomeruli are similar in IDDM and NIDDM. Nephropathy is related to the duration of the diabetes occurring in around one-half of patients where the onset of diabetes has been before the age of 30 and the duration has been more than 30 years (Watkins 1982). Nephropathy in older patients with NIDDM has not been so carefully studied.

It is likely that of patients developing diabetes at the age 60 years or more, only some 1% will die in renal failure. Cardiovascular death is much more likely. The earliest sign of nephropathy in both IDDM and NIDDM is the presence of micro-albuminuria. This is a powerful predictor of the development of fixed proteinuria (greater than 500 mg/24 h-Albustix positive) and of mortality, usually from cardiovascular causes (Mogensen 1984). Microalbuminuria may be detected at presentation, as occasionally may be fixed proteinuria. This so-called silent phase is then followed by intermittent Albustix positive proteinuria, and finally fixed proteinuria. This heralds the onset of a gradual and progressive decline in renal function, leading to end-stage renal disease after an average of 7 years. The progression of nephropathy is often accompanied by hypertension. As the serum albumin falls and renal function deteriorates, there is progressive fluid retention with peripheral oedema and pulmonary congestion. Following this, symptoms of uraemia develop.

In old age, the effects of diabetes on renal function have to be distinguished from those of ageing, and treatment with diuretics. There is the further complication that changes in creatine production in old people limit the validity of the serum creatinine and the creatinine clearance test as indices of renal function (Hodkinson 1977). One approach is to calculate the glomerular filtration rate from a nomogram which takes into account body weight and serum urea and creatinine concentrations (Denham et al. 1975).

Other complications of diabetes are almost always present, and indeed the absence of any evidence of diabetic retinopathy in a diabetic patient with proteinuria raises the question of whether the renal pathology is unrelated to diabetes and whether renal biopsy may be necessary. The latter should only be performed, however, if there is convincing evidence that a positive diagnosis will determine an important change in the management of a patient particularly if he or she is elderly.

Diabetics may also develop renal impairment as a result of chronic pyelonephritis. This can be difficult to diagnose as the systemic effects and localising signs of UTI are masked by both ageing and diabetes. It may thus present as a feeling of malaise, an episode of confusion, or a deterioration in diabetic control, and in these circumstances a mid-stream specimen of urine should be sent for culture. Patients with autonomic neuropathy frequently suffer from incomplete voiding and may be prone to recurrent urinary infection.

One of the most serious renal disorders in diabetes is renal papillary necrosis (Eknoyan et al. 1982). The risk of this is increased in patients on non-steroidal anti-inflammatory agents. It is also often associated with an episode of acute pyelonephritis. Whatever the cause, the basic lesion is that of ischaemia in the renal papillae. It presents with the clinical features of impaired renal function associated with gross or microscopic haematuria. More detailed examination of the urine may reveal the presence of sloughed papillary fragments. Colicky lumbar or ureteric pain is also common but, as is often the case in old age, symptoms may be atypical with no pyrexia or loin pain. Excretory urography shows characteristic changes, but these are not always present, and the investigation is hazardous if there is severe azotaemia.

Osteoporosis

Patients with diabetes have a reduced trabecular and cortical bone mass (Heath et al. 1980). The reason for the relationship is not clear, but the severity of osteoporosis does not increase with the duration of diabetes. Surprisingly, the reduction in bone mass in diabetics is not associated with an increased incidence of fractures. Indeed the relative risk of fractures is appreciably less in diabetics than in age and sex matched controls (Heath et al. 1980).

Skin

A number of skin disorders may occur in elderly diabetics (infections are discussed in the next section). Diabetic dermopathy may manifest as red atrophic plaques (necrobiosis lipoidica diabeticorum), particularly in the long-standing insulin-dependent diabetic patient. A characteristic bullous eruption (bullosis diabeticorum) may occur on the hands and feet of diabetic patients. The aetiology of this is unclear but neuropathy, micro-angiopathy and hypoglycaemia may be precipitating factors.

Infections

Diabetic patients have an increased susceptibility to infection. Factors responsible for this include impaired lymphocyte function presenting as impaired cell-mediated immunity and abnormalities of neutrophil function (Wilson 1986).

Ageing itself is accompanied by a wide spectrum of changes in immunological and phagocytic activity (Fox 1984). These include an impairment in cell-mediated immunity, a reduced antibody response to foreign antigens, and defective neutrophil chemotaxis, phagocytosis and antimicrobial activity.

Not only do the effects of ageing and diabetes increase the risk and severity of infections, they also mask many of the features of an infection such as pyrexia, leucocytosis and focal signs, so that the condition goes unrecognised.

The range and sites of infections in elderly diabetic patients are legion (Sen and Louria 1983).

Skin

Diabetic patients of all ages are susceptible to boils, carbuncles and cellulitis. Skin sepsis is particularly dangerous in patients with neuropathy or a poor peripheral circulation. Thus a minor foot infection may rapidly spread to cause fasciitis, osteomyelitis or septicaemia. Local or spreading gangrene may also occur. Indirect signs of fasciitis are a smooth shiny blistered overlying skin, and systemic effects such as fever, malaise or even a diffuse intravascular coagulation defect.

In a micro-biological study of diabetic skin lesions an average of 3.3 organisms per swab were isolated. Over one-third of the organisms were gram-positive cocci, mainly *Staphylococcus aureus*. One-quarter of the strains were coliforms. Anaerobic organisms were isolated from 10% of the swabs (Jones et al. 1985).

Necrotising fascial infections in sites other than the foot also occur, particularly affecting the abdominal wall and perineum. While they can occur spontaneously, they are often associated with surgery or trauma. They are associated with much morbidity and significant mortality. More common infecting organisms are streptococci, staphylococci, *Klebsiella*, *Bacteroides* and *Escherichia coli*.

Ear

Elderly diabetic patients may present with a particularly severe otitis externa. This is associated with a purulent discharge and there is swelling and tenderness around the ear. The infection is caused by *Pseudomonas aeruginosa* and spreads to surrounding tissues, so that there may be features of a mastoid infection and compression of the facial nerve. Once fully established, the condition carries a high mortality.

Gastro-intestinal Tract

The most common gastro-intestinal infection in this situation is mucocutaneous candidiasis, presenting as white patches on the tongue which, if removed, leave bleeding raw areas. Occasionally the condition spreads to involve the oesophagus giving rise to a painful dysphagia, and producing characteristic radiological abnormalities if a barium swallow is performed. In patients with a diabetic autonomic neuropathy, reduced small bowel peristalsis may result in ileal over-growth by colonic micro-organisms with severe episodic diarrhoea and faecal incontinence.

Urogenital Tract

There is an increased incidence of urinary tract infections in diabetic women but not in men. In one study, 19% of women had a urinary tract infection (Forland et al. 1977). Initially, only 43% of infections involved the renal parenchyma, but after 7 weeks the figure had risen to 79%. This suggests that, in diabetes, the infection starts in the bladder and later ascends to the kidneys. No figures are available for the incidence of urinary infections in elderly diabetics, but coincidental disorders such as a neurogenic bladder, cystocele, prostatic enlargement, or long-term catheterisation are likely to make this high in both men and women.

A reduced resistance to infection means that elderly patients are more likely to suffer severe complications from pyelonephritis. The problem of renal papillary necrosis has already been discussed. Another is a perinephric abscess. This may present with fever, flank tenderness and rigors, but the effects of age and diabetes on immunological function may mask these and the only manifestations may be lethargy, malaise or confusion. Only 75% of patients have organisms in their urine so that a negative culture of this does not exclude the diagnosis.

NIDDM often presents in women as vaginal candidiasis characterised by itch, erythema and multiple white patches. Fungi are sometimes grown in urine samples, but these are usually contaminants, and serious renal parenchymal involvement is rare.

Respiratory System

Elderly diabetics who develop influenza have an increased mortality over their non-diabetic contemporaries (Schoenbaum 1979). It is also likely that their diabetes increases the risk of developing a bronchopneumonia, but the evidence for this is conflicting (Sen and Louria 1983).

It is also unlikely that NIDDM is associated with an increased incidence of pulmonary tuberculosis, but diabetes may predispose to the reactivation of tuberculosis, and once the infection has occurred it is more likely to be severe and more likely to involve an unusual site such as a lower lobe.

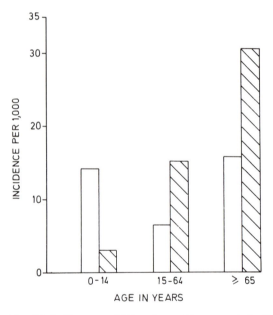

Fig. 4.3. Incidence per 1000 patients of bacteraemia in diabetic (*hatched bars*) and non-diabetic patients. (After Bryan et al. 1985.)

Bacteraemia

Diabetes doubles the risk of elderly patients developing a bacteraemia (Bryan et al. 1985) (Fig. 4.3). In a recent study over a 2-year period, one-third of bacteraemic episodes occurred in patients with long-standing diabetes, the commonest source being the urinary tract (MacFarlane et al. 1986). It was noted that elderly patients were frequently apyrexial despite being bacteraemic. Common infecting organisms include *Staphylococcus aureus, Klebsiella* and *Proteus mirabilis*. While septicaemia, particularly gram-negative septicaemia, causes a high mortality, this is no greater in diabetic than non-diabetic patients.

Acute Metabolic Imbalance

Diabetic Ketoacidosis

This condition is particularly common in young diabetics with insulin-dependent diabetes, most series giving a mean age of occurrence of between 30 and 40 years (Biegelman 1971). In a large survey in Nottingham, 26% of patients presenting with severe uncontrolled diabetes were over the age of 60 years. In this group the mortality was 47%. Three-quarters had significant ketoacidosis (standard bicarbonate less than or equal to 15 mmol/l), and the other quarter hyperglycaemic, hyperosmolar non-ketotic coma.

Impaired homeostatic control and an increased prevalence of cardiovascular disease account for the increased mortality in elderly patients. In an autopsy series of 30 of the patients from Nottingham, uncontrolled diabetes was the only cause of death found in two-thirds of the patients, but with increasing age severe hypotension and hypothermia were adverse prognostic factors. The majority of deaths from diabetic ketoacidosis were in the first 48 h in contrast with hyperglycaemic non-ketotic patients, in whom deaths occurred later and were due to thrombolic disorders in pneumonia (Gale et al. 1981).

Non-ketotic Hyperglycaemic Hyperosmolar Coma

This condition occurs almost exclusively in elderly non-insulin-dependent diabetics, when it may be the presenting feature of the condition. In this situation there is a relative insulin deficiency but enough residual activity to prevent lipolysis and hepatic ketogenesis so that there is little ketoacidosis.

The disorder is preceded in about one-half of cases by stress such as infection, surgery, stroke or myocardial infarction (McCurdy 1970).

Progress of the illness is slow and patients may be ill up to 14 days prior to presentation, much longer than is typically seen for diabetic ketoacidosis. As the hyperglycaemia progresses (sometimes worsened by glucose-rich drinks in patients not known to be diabetics), the inevitable osmotic diuresis causes dehydration. Commencement of treatment with diuretics, even in modest doses, may also set in course the sequence of events leading to severe hyperglycaemia (Fonseca and Phear 1982), and exacerbate dehydration. As renal perfusion decreases, further glucose retention occurs.

The condition develops insidiously and the level of consciousness of the patient diminishes as the plasma osmolality rises. There is considerable individual variation, however, and in a patient with a serum osmolality of 380 mosmol/kg the level of consciousness might vary from drowsy to comatose (Gill and Alberti 1985a). Dehydration is often of sufficient severity to cause hypotension and shock, and this in turn may embarrass an already compromised coronary artery perfusion. The problems of identifying dehydration are discussed elsewhere (Chap. 9).

Hyperglycaemia and ageing may suppress hypothalamic function, so that the patient may not feel thirsty and this may be one of the reasons why severe dehydration appears insidiously in this disorder (Greene 1986). As the condition progresses the patient may present a wide range of focal neurological signs including focal and generalised convulsions, hemiparesis, extensor plantar responses, nystagmus and visual hallucinations (Grant and Warlow 1985). These are the results of metabolic derangement rather than vascular damage, and can be reversed by controlling the hyperglycaemia.

Investigation reveals that there is glycosuria but ketones are absent from the urine, or present in only small amounts. The blood glucose concentration is increased, usually in the region of 40–60 mmol/l, although levels as high as 250 mmol/l have been recorded. By definition, tests of acid–base balance are near normal. The blood urea and creatinine concentrations are elevated, but the serum sodium concentration though often increased may be normal or low. The latter may be due to the osmotic effect of severe hyperglycaemia (Gill and Alberti 1985a).

The serum osmolality is high by definition and may be calculated by the equation $2(Na^+ + K^+)$ + glucose + urea (all in mmol/l). Accordingly it is the marked elevation in glucose and urea which usually contributes more to the hyperosmolality than the elevated serum sodium. Hyperosmolality and dehydration cause a rise in the haemoglobin concentration with an increase in the viscosity and coagulability of the blood, so that there is a high incidence of syndromes associated with arterial or venous thrombosis or thrombo-embolism. This accounts, in part, for a mortality rate of between 40% and 70%. A further factor in this is that the presentation is gradual and undramatic, so that the condition often remains untreated until a late stage in its evolution.

In some elderly patients, particularly those with significant infection, a mixed picture develops in which there is both severe hyperosmolality and a degree of ketoacidosis.

The presenting condition itself such as myocardial infarction, may carry a poor prognosis. In the Nottingham series, among patients aged 50 years or older, the death rate was 38% for DKA, and 58% for hyperglycaemic, non-ketotic coma while, in 65% of the patients presenting with hyperglycaemic non-ketotic coma, diabetes was previously undiagnosed (Gale et al. 1981).

Lactic Acidosis

Mechanisms of lactic acidosis likely to be operative in elderly patients include hypoxia (from any cause, e.g. heart failure or respiratory failure), a decrease in the hepatic removal of lactate (e.g. in liver disease) or poisoning by mitochondrial toxins (e.g. biguanides). The situation in the elderly diabetic is particularly complex since a number of factors may co-exist including hypoxic states, hepatic impairment, the diabetes itself, and the use of hypoglycaemic agents. These all interact to precipitate lactic acidosis.

The drug most frequently implicated as a major cause of lactic acidosis is the biguanide oral hypoglycaemic agent, phenformin. Though the precise mode of action is uncertain, it probably involves interference with the lactic acid transport mechanism in the mitochondrial membrane. All biguanides cause a mild hyperlacticaemia in normal use. The incidence of lactic acidosis in diabetics on phenformin is around 1 per 1000. Buformin, another biguanide, causes the condition less frequently while metformin is rarely a factor (Luft et al. 1978). Phenformin and buformin should no longer be used.

The mortality from lactic acidosis is around 50% and is increased with age, cardiac disease, and renal or hepatic impairment. When metformin is used, lactic acidosis can be avoided if the drug is not used (a) in above recommended doses, (b) in patients with renal insufficiency when metformin clearance is reduced, (c) in patients with liver disease and (d) in patients with heart failure.

Lactic acidosis should be suspected in patients presenting with the signs of metabolic acidosis – hyperventilation, tachycardia, vasodilatation, hypotension and clouding of consciousness. Dehydration is not usually a problem. If the patient is a diabetic, and taking a biguanide, the blood glucose is only marginally elevated, and urinary and plasma ketone concentrations are not detected in significant amounts. The serum biochemistry reveals a marked anion gap $[(Na^+ + K^+) - (Cl^- \ HCO_3^-)]$ often greater than 25 mmol/l, while arterial blood gas analysis reveals a low pH (usually less than 7.2), a low pCO_2 and a low standard bicarbonate with a significant base deficit. The osmolality is usually normal. Plasma lactate concentrations are always elevated above 7 mmol/l and usually much higher (Gill and Alberti 1985b).

References

Andres R (1971) Effect of age in interpretation of glucose and tolbutamide tolerance tests. In: Fajans SS, Sussman KE (eds) Diabetes mellitus: diagnosis and treatment, vol. 3. American Diabetes Association, pp 115–120

Biegelman PM (1971) Severe ketoacidosis (Diabetic "coma"): 482 episodes in 257 patients; experience of 3 years. Diabetes 20: 490–500

Brierley JB (1976) Cerebral hypoxia. In: Blackwood W, Corsellis JAN (eds) Greenfield's Neuropathology, 3rd edn. Edward Arnold, London, pp 43–85

Bron AJ, Cheng H (1986) Cataract and retinopathy: screening for treatable retinopathy. Clin Endocrinol Metab 15: 971–999

Bryan CS, Reynolds KL, Metzger WI (1985) Bacteraemia in diabetic patients: comparison of incidence and mortality with non-diabetic patients. Diabetes Care 8: 244–249

Butterfield WJH (1964) The Bedford diabetes survey. Proc R Soc Med 57: 196–200

Campbell DR, Hoar CS, Wheecock FC (1984) Carotid artery surgery in diabetes patients. Arch Surg 119: 1405–1407

De Fronzo RA, Ferrannini E (1987) Regulation of hepatic glucose metabolism in humans. Diabetes Metab Rev 3: 415–459

Denham MJ, Hodkinson HM, Fisher M (1975) Glomerular filtration rate in sick elderly inpatients. Age Ageing 4: 32–36

Dyck PJ, Hansen S, Kames J et al. (1985) Capillary number and percentage closed in human diabetic nerve. Proc Natl Acad Sci USA 82: 2513–2517

Edmonds ME (1986) The diabetic foot. Pathophysiology and treatment. Clin Endocrinol Metab 15: 889–916

Eknoyan G, Quribi W, Grissom RT et al. (1982) Renal papillary necrosis: an update. Medicine 61: 55–73

Ewing DJ, Clarke BF (1982) Diagnosis and management of diabetic autonomic neuropathy. Br Med J 285: 916–918

Fonseca V, Phear DN (1982) Hyperosmolar non-ketotic diabetic syndrome precipitated by treatment with diuretics. Br Med J 284: 36–37

Forland M, Thomas V, Shelokov A (1977) Urinary tract infections in patients with diabetes mellitus. Studies on antibody coating of bacteria. JAMA 238: 1924–1926

Fox RA (1984) Immunology and infection in the elderly. Churchill Livingstone, London

Gale EAM, Dornan TL, Tattersall RB (1981) Severe uncontrolled diabetes in the over 50's. Diabetologia 21: 25–28

Garcia MJ, McNamara PM, Gordon T et al. (1974) Morbidity and mortality in diabetics in the Framingham population. Sixteen year follow-up study. Diabetes 23: 105–111

Gill GV, Alberti KGMM (1985a) Hyperosmolar non-ketotic coma. Practical Diabetes 2: 30–35

Gill GV, Alberti KGMM (1985b) Lactic acidosis. Practical Diabetes 2: 15–19

Grant C, Warlow CP (1985) Focal epilepsy in diabetic non-ketotic hyperglycaemia. Bri Med J 290: 1204–1205

Greene DA (1986) Acute and chronic complications of diabetes mellitus in older patients. Am J Med 80 (Suppl 5a): 39–53

Hayford JT, Weydert JA, Thompson RG (1983) Validity of urine glucose measurements for estimating plasma glucose concentration. Diabetes Care 6: 40–44

Heath H, Melton LJ, Chu CP (1980) Diabetes mellitus and risk of skeletal fracture. N Engl J Med 303: 567–570

Hodkinson HM (1977) Biochemical diagnosis of the elderly. Chapman and Hall, London

Jarrett RJ (1985) The Whitehall Study. Practical Diabetes 2: 97–100

Jones EW, Edwards R, Finch R (1985) A microbiological study of diabetic foot lesions. Diabetic Med 2: 213–215

Jung R (1984) Endocrinological aspects of obesity. Clin Endocrinol Metab 13: 597–612

Karasik A, Modan M, Hallen H et al. (1984) Senile cataract and glucose intolerance: the Israel study of glucose intolerance, obesity and hypertension (the Israel GOH study). Diabetes Care 7: 52–56

Keen H, Ng Tang Fui S (1982) The definition and classification of diabetes mellitus. Clin Endocrinol Metab 11: 279–305

Kent S (1976) Is diabetes a form of accelerated ageing? Geriatrics 31: 140–151

Kilvert A, Fitzgerald MG, Wright AD, Nattrass M (1984) Newly diagnosed insulin dependent diabetes mellitus in elderly patients. Diabetic Med 1: 115–118

Kolterman OG (1987) The impact of sulphonylureas on hepatic glucose metabolism in type II diabetes. Diabetes Metab Rev 3: 399–414

Kreines, Johnson E, Albrink M et al. (1985) The cause of peripheral vascular disease in non-insulin dependent diabetes. Diabetes Care 8: 235–243

Luft D, Schmulling RM, Eggstein M (1978) Lactic acidosis in biguanide-treated diabetics: a review of 330 cases. Diabetologia 14: 75–87

MacFarlane IA, Brown RM, Bibdon DW, Fitzgerald MG (1986) Bacteraemia in diabetes. J Infect 12: 213–219

McCurdy DK (1970) Hyperosmolar hyperglycaemic non-ketotic diabetic coma. Med Clin N Am 54: 683–699

Modan M, Halkin H, Almeg S et al. (1985) A link between hypertension, obesity and glucose intolerance. J Clin Invest 75: 809–817

Mogenson CE (1984) Microalbuminuria predicts clinical proteinaemia and early mortality in maturity onset diabetes. New Engl J Med 311: 89–93

Morris DV, Nabarro JDN (1984) Pancreatic cancer and diabetes mellitus. Diabetic Med 1: 119–121

Ohlson LO, Larsson B, Svardsudd K et al. (1985) The influence of body fat distribution on the incidence of diabetes mellitus. 13.5 years of follow-up of the participants in the study of men born in 1913. Diabetes 34: 1055–1058

O'Rahilly SP, Nugent Z, Redonski AS et al. (1986) Beta cell dysfunction rather than insulin insensitivity is the primary defect in familial type 2 diabetes. Lancet 2: 360–363

Perlmuter LC, Hakami MK, Hodgson-Harrington C et al. (1984) Decreased cognitive function in ageing non-insulin dependent diabetic patients. Am J Med 77: 1043–1048

Petri MP, Gatling W, Petri LM, Hill RD (1986) Diabetes in the elderly – an epidemiological perspective. Practical Diabetes 3: 153–155

Pyke DA (1979) Diabetes: The genetic connections. Diabetologia 17: 333–343

Pyorala K, Laabsor M, Vusitupa M (1987) Diabetes and atherosclerosis: an epidemiological view. Diabetes Metab Rev 3: 463–524

Schoenbaum SC (1979) How to minimise complications of diabetes. Geriatrics 34 (March): 51–61

Segal P, Triester G, Sandak R et al. (1984) The prevalence of diabetic retinopathy: effect of sex, age, duration of disease, and mode of therapy. Diabetes Care 6: 149–151

Sen P, Louria DB (1983) Infectious complications in the elderly diabetic patient. Geriatrics 38 (February): 63–66, 71–72

Suarez L, Barrett-Conner E (1984) Interaction between cigarette smoking and diabetes mellitus – the prediction of death attributed to cardiovascular disease. Am J Epidemiol 120: 670–675

Tattersall RB (1984) Diabetes in the elderly – a neglected area. Diabetiologia 27: 167–173

Vracko R (1982) A comparison of the microvascular lesions in diabetes with those of normal ageing. J Am Geriatr Soc 30: 201–205

Vranic M, Berger M (1979) Exercise and diabetes mellitus. Diabetes 28: 147–167

Ward JD (1982) The diabetic leg. Diabetologia 22: 141–147

Ward WK, Beard JC, Porte D (1986) Clinical aspects of islet β-cell function in non-insulin dependent diabetes mellitus. Diabetes Metab Rev 2: 297–313

Watkins PJ (1982) ABC of diabetes. Nephropathy. Br Med J 285: 627–628

Wilkinson DG (1981) Psychiatric aspects of diabetes mellitus. Br J Psychiatry 138: 1–9

Williams TJ (1981) Diabetes mellitus. Clin Endocrinol Metab 10: 179–194

Wilson PW, Anderson KM, Kannel WB (1986) Epidemiology of diabetes mellitus in the elderly. The Framingham Study. Am J Med 80 (suppl 5a): 3–9

Wilson RM (1986) Neutrophil function in diabetes. Diabetic Medicine 3: 509–512

Zimmet P (1982) Type 2 (non-insulin-dependent) diabetes – an epidemiological overview. Diabetologia 22: 399–411

5 Diabetes Mellitus: Management

The treatment of diabetes in the elderly differs from that in the young in that there is much more emphasis on the management of the non-insulin-dependent (NIDD) patients. There also is the issue of the extent to which the prevention of long-term complications should outweigh immediate convenience in patients with a limited life expectancy. Consideration also has to be given to the effects which ageing and disease have upon the metabolism, excretion and end-organ responses to hypoglycaemic agents. Finally, there may be problems of ensuring compliance with treatment in mentally and physically frail individuals. They may have greater difficulty than younger patients in understanding the nature and management of diabetes, and using such techniques as the self-monitoring of blood glucose levels.

Aims of Treatment

Allowing for the differing circumstances of individuals the following aims of management are generally applicable to elderly patients: (1) relief from symptoms of hyperglycaemia, (2) avoidance of hypoglycaemia and (3) avoidance of complications where possible and rapid detection and treatment if these do occur. Some consideration should also be given to avoidance of diabetic hyperglycaemic decompensation during intercurrent illness.

Clearcut guidelines for controlling the blood glucose level are not practicable, but maintaining post-prandial blood glucose levels at less than 12 mmol/l should ensure that the patient is free from symptoms of hyperglycaemia, and in the absence of symptoms it may be permissible to allow an elderly patient to run a higher blood glucose than this. A post-prandial blood glucose of less than 6 mmol/l in a patient on a sulphonylurea or insulin usually means that there is a risk of hypoglycaemia.

Diet

A dietary history will reveal which aspects of the patient's diet may need particular attention. Has the patient been consuming large quantities of lemonade because of thirst? What scope is there for a reduction in total energy intake in an obese patient? How active or sedentary is the elderly person and what will be his energy requirements in relation to this? What kinds of food is the patient used to eating and is he likely to be the kind of individual who will make major changes to this on medical advice?

A patient near ideal weight requires a weight-maintaining diet which avoids simple sugars, while an obese patient needs a reducing diet in which the total energy intake for both fat and carbohydrate is reduced.

In recent years there has been much discussion on the appropriate carbohydrate and fat contents of diabetic diets and patients have been encouraged to increase the carbohydrate proportion of their diets to at least 50% of total energy intake, the carbohydrate being taken as complex carbohydrates and not simple sugars. The corresponding reduction in saturated fat has been recommended to reduce the risk of atherosclerosis. Much has also been written about the role of various forms of dietary fibre. Fibre-rich diets high in complex carbohydrates can improve insulin sensitivity, thus reducing post-prandial glycaemia and improving plasma lipid profiles. These diets have, however, received relatively little evaluation in elderly patients living in the community. It may well be that any major departure from traditional eating habits will be rejected by such individuals as unsuited to their lifestyles.

A diet prescribed for an elderly patient should be explained in terms which will be familiar to both him and his family. The efficacy of this approach has been described by Wilson et al. (1980). If someone else in the household is responsible for food preparation, it is important that that person should be interviewed by the dietician. Attention should also be given to whether the patient has Meals on Wheels or eats at a senior citizens' lunch club. It is also important that any dietary advice is not deemed "too expensive" by the patient and thus not heeded.

Patients receiving insulin should be advised on the importance of taking regular meals and a bed-time snack to avoid nocturnal hypoglycaemia. Old people, however, are likely to have problems learning a carbohydrate exchange system based on the metric measures, and it is unrealistic to expect them to weigh food portions.

A useful, though minor, adjunct to dietary restriction is to increase physical activity. There is evidence that this produces an improvement in tissue sensitivity to insulin which is independent of weight loss. This is obviously only practicable in a patient who is not incapacitated by locomotor, neurological or cardiorespiratory disease.

Oral Hypoglycaemic Agents

Depending on the strictness of criteria of glycaemic control many elderly patients can be effectively treated by dietary measures alone (Wilson et al. 1980). It is only where these have failed after an appropriate duration of trial (at least 3 months unless the patient has marked symptoms of hyperglycaemia), that oral hypo-glycaemic agents should be introduced. Prior to resorting to these, compliance with dietary advice should be reviewed. Patients should also be instructed that drugs are only an adjunct to other measures and are unlikely to provide adequate control unless there are dietary modifications.

Sulphonylureas

The precise mode of action of the sulphonylureas is unclear despite their use for almost 30 years, but it seems likely that they both stimulate the secretion of insulin in response to hyperglycaemia, and reduce the resistance of peripheral tissues to the effect of insulin on glucose utilisation. Recent studies have demonstrated in vivo and in vitro effects of sulphonylurea drugs on insulin action at both receptor and post-receptor sites (Kolterman 1987). Whatever their mode of action, they are as effective in elderly as in younger diabetics (Martin and Kesson 1986).

A wide range of both first- and second-generation agents is now available but in old age a prime consideration is the duration of action of a drug (Peden et al. 1983). Those with prolonged action are likely to cause accumulation with resultant hypoglycaemia. There is the converse problem that patients may have difficulty in remembering to take a tablet several times a day. Even here, however, the conse-quences of omitting one tablet taken three times a day are likely to be less serious than those of omitting one tablet taken once a day. Individual choice may also be influenced by the route of elimination of a drug and whether the patient has clinical or biochemical evidence of renal or hepatic impairment. The route of elimination, duration of action, daily dose range and number of doses per day of commonly used sulphonylureas are listed in Table 5.1. Their half-lives are not listed because these have little bearing on the duration of their hypoglycaemic effects.

Table 5.1. Route of elimination, duration of action, daily dose range and number of doses per day of commonly used sulphonylureas (Jackson and Bressler 1981a, b)

Agent	Route elimination	Duration of action (h)	Daily dose range	Doses per day
Tolbutamide	Liver metabolism	6–10	0.5–2 g	2–3
Chlorpropamide	Liver metabolism	24–72	100–500 mg	1
Acetohexamide	Renal excretion of active metabolites	8–12	0.25–1.5 g	2
Tolazamide	Liver metabolism	12–18	100–1000 mg	1–2
Glibenclamide	Liver metabolism	16+	2.5–15 mg	1–2
Glipizide	Liver metabolism	>6	2.5–20 mg	1–2
Gliclazide	Liver metabolism	6–12	80–240 mg	1–2
Glymidine	Liver metabolism Renal excretion of active metabolites	4–8	0.5–2 g	2–3
Glibornuride	Liver metabolism	8–10	4–50 mg	1–2
Gliquidone	Liver metabolism	4–8	15–180 mg	1–3

Table 5.2. Drugs potentiating the hypoglycaemic effect of sulphonylureas (Jackson and Bressler 1981a, b)

Drug	Mechanism
Alcohol	Decreased gluconeogenesis
Salicylates	Increased insulin release
Coumarin anticoagulants	Decreased hepatic metabolism of sulphonylureas
Beta-adrenergic blockers	Decreased glyconeogenesis

Note: Many other drugs less commonly used in old people cause similar interactions.

The most important side effect of all the sulphonylureas is hypoglycaemia (Jackson and Bressler 1981a, b). This results in coma in around 1% of patients treated, which in turn is fatal in around 10% of cases. That this is a particular problem in old age is illustrated by a finding that 90% of patients with sulphonylurea induced hypoglycaemic coma were over the age of 60 (Berger 1971). Factors increasing the risk of this include renal and hepatic impairment. There is also the fact that elderly patients are more likely than younger patients to be taking a sulphonylurea drug, so that a greater proportion are exposed to the risk of side-effects. A sudden reduction in food intake and unaccustomed exertion are also important. There are also several groups of drugs which interact with sulphonylureas to increase the severity of hypoglycaemia (Table 5.2). The clinical effect of such interactions is often trivial. An example is that beta-adrenoceptor blockers cause more problems by masking the autonomic manifestations of hypoglycaemia than by potentiating its severity (Chap. 11).

Patients on sulphonylurea drugs seem less knowledgeable about hypoglycaemia than patients on insulin and patients over the age of 70 are particularly uncertain (Mutch and Dingwall-Fordyce 1985). While chlorpropamide is the sulphonurea which has been most implicated in severe hypoglycaemia, glibenclamide also causes this and can stimulate further insulin release each time the blood glucose rises over a prolonged period of time. Patients may require intravenous glucose for 2 or even 3 days to control the problem. Hypoglycaemia, though less common with other sulphonylureas, still remains a potential problem with all these drugs in elderly patients.

There is the more controversial issue of whether treatment with sulphonylureas increases cardiovascular mortality. The results of the University Group Diabetes Programme in the USA which reported a significant excess of cardiac mortality in patients taking tolbutamide have proved controversial and have not been widely accepted outside the USA. They have nonetheless been responsible for a reappraisal of the role of drugs and diet in the management of NIDDM (Jackson and Bressler 1981a, b). If the drugs have an effect on cardiovascular mortality it is unclear whether this is because of increased atherogenesis or from an arrhythmogenic effect.

Sulphonylureas should be considered for use in patients with diabetes whose blood glucose concentration has not been adequately controlled by diet alone. As a rough guide, patients inadequately treated by a diet who have random plasma glucose levels between 11 and 20 mmol/l should be treated in this way. Those with levels over this may well need insulin. Treatment with sulphonylureas is associated with weight gain, a particular problem in patients who are often already obese.

The first generation agent tolbutamide is particularly useful in elderly patients. It has a relatively short duration of action (6–12 h) and is given before meals twice or three times daily. It can be initiated in a dose of 500 mg twice daily, gradually increasing this to a maximum of 2 g per day. There is no evidence that any one sulphonylurea has greater efficacy than another although second generation drugs are more potent on a weight-for-weight basis. Nonetheless, some patients do appear to respond better to one drug than another and it is worthwhile trying a second generation drug if tolbutamide fails. In view of the risk of prolonged hypoglycaemia, it is unwise to initiate treatment with chlorpropamide or glibenclamide in patients over the age of 70, especially if they have renal impairment. Many patients well controlled on these drugs survive into old age, and it is then necessary to review their continued use. Particular attention should be paid to actively questioning such patients about symptoms suggesting episodes of mild hypoglycaemia.

Tolbutamide like chlorpropamide may cause water retention and hyponatraemia, a potential problem in patients with heart failure. Second generation drugs do not have this side-effect.

If a second generation sulphonylurea drug is to be tried then the shorter-acting agents gliquidone, glipizide or gliclazide appear to be most appropriate. If a sulphonylurea causes a rash, then glymidine, a sulphapyrimidine drug, may be tried.

Treatment with any of the shorter-acting sulphonylurea drugs should start with the minimum recommended dose, increasing this twice weekly until effective control is achieved or until it becomes clear that the drug is ineffective. Generally the best results are obtained with patients who respond to small doses. If, some time after the diabetes has been stabilised, there is further deterioration, secondary problems such as a urinary tract infection should be excluded. It is also wise to review dietary compliance, particularly if weight gain has occurred. There may be scope for increasing the dose of sulphonylurea, but this is rarely effective for long and secondary drug failures occur at a rate of 5% per annum. A biguanide may be added to the sulphonylurea therapy at this stage, but the efficacy of this manoeuvre has been questioned (Nattrass 1986).

Biguanides

The mode of action of these drugs is unclear. They have an anorectic effect, and cause a degree of malabsorption. They are, however, only hypoglycaemic in the presence of insulin and there is evidence that they increase the sensitivity of peripheral tissues to the hypoglycaemic action of insulin, perhaps by an effect on insulin receptors. A major advantage over the sulphonylureas is that although they reduce blood glucose levels, they do not stimulate insulin secretion, so that they do not cause hypoglycaemia. An important effect is to inhibit gluconeogenesis in the liver at a mitochondrial level, causing accumulation of gluconeogenic precursors and inducing mild hyperlactataemia (Bailey 1988).

The only biguanide in common use is metformin. This has a slow and variable pattern of absorption, is eliminated entirely by the kidneys and has a half-life of

2–4 h. If there is renal impairment accumulation does occur. The risk of this, however, is not hypoglycaemia but that it may play a part in the development of lactic acidosis.

The most common side-effects are anorexia, vomiting and diarrhoea. In obese elderly diabetics, anorexia can be a positive advantage in that this, coupled with a catabolic effect, promotes weight loss. Diarrhoea is more troublesome and occurs in around 20% of patients (Dandona et al. 1983). In frail old people with limited mobility or a lax anal sphincter this may result in faecal incontinence. Another problem is that biguanides may reduce the absorption of vitamin B_{12} from the terminal ileum, so that regular checks of serum B_{12} levels are advisable. There is some evidence that if metformin is given after meals and the dose increased gradually, it is better tolerated.

The problem which has given rise to most debate is that of lactic acidosis (Campbell 1984). Phenformin has frequently been implicated but surveillance in Sweden, the United Kingdom and Canada suggests that if metformin is used the risk of this is negligible (Table 5.3). The only proviso is that the drug should not be given to patients with impaired renal function, liver disease or severe cardio-respiratory disease.

The approach to treatment with metformin is essentially that for sulphonylureas in that it should be started at its lowest dose of 500 mg daily increasing this gradually to 2.0 g daily or until optimal control has been achieved. The main indication for use is an adjunct to diet in obese patients.

Table 5.3. Incidence of lactic acidosis in patients treated with metformin in Sweden, United Kingdom and Canada (Campbell 1984)

Country	No of cases	Size of population (patient years)
Sweden	7	83 500
United Kingdom	0	330 000
Canada	0	56 000

Guar

There has been considerable interest in the use of guar gum to reduce post-prandial hyperglycaemia. Various preparations have been used but all suffer problems with palatability and intestinal side effects are frequent. Results in terms of improvement in glycaemic control have been generally disappointing and it appears that if guar is to have any useful effect then it must be intimately mixed with food (Fuessel et al. 1986). Guar is therefore unlikely to be a useful adjunct to therapy in the elderly diabetic.

Other approaches to the manipulation of carbohydrate and hence glucose absorption from the gut include the use of experimental drugs which inhibit alpha-glucosidase enzymes in the small intestine.

Insulin

Indication for Treatment

Insulin is clearly indicated if a patient presents with diabetic ketoacidosis (DKA) or hyperglycaemic hyperosmolar non-ketotic coma, although in this case the need for insulin may only be temporary. Patients presenting with marked weight loss or significant ketonuria should also be treated with insulin, and those who have failed to respond to combined oral hypoglycaemic therapy should be considered for insulin therapy. In an obese patient, however, it is wise to review compliance with diet and drugs before switching to insulin. An explanation of the implications of insulin injection therapy may make such patients more compliant with diet and oral treatment. In one study of elderly obese diabetics with poor glycaemic control on insulin therapy, a combined in-patient and out-patient programme emphasising diet resulted in significant weight loss in the majority of patients, so that insulin could be discontinued (Reaven 1985). Painful peripheral neuropathy or amyotrophy may also be an indication for achieving tighter glycaemic control with insulin. Finally, some patients require insulin when an infected foot ulcer or other insult destabilises control. If an infection precipitates diabetic ketoacidosis in a patient or oral agents then it may well be possible to re-introduce the previous therapy when the acute situation has resolved. Patients on diet or diet plus oral hypoglycaemic agent also need insulin during major surgery. Many centres now also treat such patients with insulin during management of an acute myocardial infarction, although the benefits are as yet unproven.

Physicians are often reluctant to submit elderly patients to insulin therapy. There is no doubt, however, that non-obese patients poorly controlled on oral hypoglycaemic agents experience a considerable improvement in their sense of well-being when improved glycaemic control is induced by optimal insulin therapy and that this will also abolish troublesome nocturia.

Choice of Preparation

At present, major changes are occurring in the types of insulin available. Recombinant DNA techniques have provided the technology, with micro-organisms producing limitless amounts of human insulin. This has resulted in one major insulin manufacturer discontinuing purified pork insulin products in favour of human insulin, while another has recently discontinued the production of beef insulin. It is likely, therefore, that all patients requiring insulin will eventually receive human insulin. The range of human insulins available is already extensive and includes short-acting neutral soluble preparations; intermediate-acting isophane (NPH) and insulin zinc suspension (lente) preparations; and long-acting preparations (ultralente). In addition, a variety of mixtures of short and intermediate-acting insulins are available.

In terms of efficacy there appears to be little difference between purified pork insulins and their human equivalents. There is some evidence that genetically engineered human insulins may be rather faster in onset of action than the purified pork preparations. It is, therefore, rather surprising that there have been anecdotal reports that patients may lose their normal warning symptoms of hypoglycaemia on transfer from pork to human insulins (Teuscher and Berger 1987).

Human ultralente insulin is substantially shorter in duration of action than the previous beef ultralente preparations. Beef insulin is more antigenic than human or pork insulin and many patients on beef insulin have insulin antibodies which may not bind human insulin, so that if they change from beef to human insulin, their insulin requirements decline and they may suffer hypoglycaemia. While this is not usually a problem with patients receiving 40 units per day or less, it is wise to reduce the insulin dose of patients on larger doses by 10%–20% in anticipation of decreasing requirements.

Changes in insulin preparations must be made with great care in elderly patients. In particular, those on beef insulin have often been on this for a long time, are used to a stable state of affairs, are likely to be rather inflexible in their thinking and are often unaware of the symptoms of hypoglycaemia. Every effort should be made to avoid hypoglycaemia in these patients, in whom an episode can be psychologically and physically shattering. A further problem is that some elderly and long-standing patients are on protamine zinc insulin preparations. These are particularly long-acting and there are no human equivalents. They act for 36 h or longer so that there is a carry-over effect into the day after an injection. It is particularly important to bear this in mind when initiating a new regime, so that the dose of short-acting insulin given on the first day is modified accordingly. Careful follow-up for the 6 weeks around the changeover is vital. Here the diabetes nurse specialist may be invaluable in liaising with the patient at home.

Treatment Programme

The treatment chosen is dependent upon a variety of factors including treatment goals, the severity of diabetes and the degree of compliance to be expected from the patient and his helpers (Shuman 1984). If treatment is being initiated in an out-patient then it may be simplest to give a single breakfast dose of a relatively long-acting lente or ultra lente preparation. This should initially be 12–16 units depending on the patient's weight increasing by 2–4 units every other day until fasting blood glucose levels around 7 mmol/l have been obtained. This can be assessed by home blood glucose monitoring by the patient or carer under the supervision of the diabetic nurse specialist or GP. Particular care should be taken to avoid hypoglycaemia in the afternoon, evening or during the night.

If this regimen results in high pre-lunch blood glucose levels, a short-acting insulin should be added. The patient or carer can pre-mix the insulin in the syringe so that there is maximum flexibility for dose adjustment. Alternatively a commercial pre-mixture of soluble and isophane insulin (e.g. Human Mixtard, Humulin M2, Actraphane) can be used, but the risk of afternoon or evening hypoglycaemia must be borne in mind. If control is inadequate on a single injection of more than 30 units per day or hypoglycaemia at night is a problem, then it is usually necessary to change to a twice-daily regimen of iosphane insulin. This was frequently necessary in one group of 32 elderly diabetics (Tattersall and Scott 1987). Usually twice-daily isophane insulin is given before breakfast and before an evening meal, giving two-thirds of the dose in the morning and one-third in the evening. Dosages are then adjusted according to the pre-tea and fasting glucose levels. If glycaemic peaks occur before lunch and during the evening, consideration should be given to using a mixture of soluble and isophane insulins.

Adverse Effects

Episodes of hypoglycaemia are far more common amongst patients on insulin than those treated with sulphonylureas. As discussed already, the avoidance and recognition of hypoglycaemia may be far from satisfactory in elderly patients. Common causes include missed meals, increased physical activity (even modest physical activity can induce hypoglycaemia in someone who is normally inactive) and overtreatment or overdosage. Old people are at increased risk from hypoglycaemia because of ageing, concomitant disease (particularly cardiovascular disease), and drugs which may mask the clinical signs of hypoglycaemia. Ageing and disease also accentuate the extent to which hypoglycaemia causes end-organ damage. It is therefore crucial that patients, their relatives and carers are all aware of symptoms of signs of hypoglycaemia and how to manage it.

A useful recent development has been the manufacture of glucagon kits to facilitate administration by subcutaneous or intramuscular injection. These can be used by relatives or carers in the event of severe hypoglycaemia. Where practicable, persons living with elderly insulin-dependent diabetics should be instructed in the use of these preparations and have them available.

Problems with insulin allergy and immunoresistance are very uncommon. Since the introduction of highly purified insulins, lipatrophy at injection sites has been rarely seen. Lipohypertrophy with fibro-fatty masses at injection sites is common and usually due to poor rotation of injection sites. Specific training in this may be helpful.

Practical Considerations in Management

Communication defects and mental impairment limit the extent to which some elderly patients can comply with dietary and therapeutic regimens. In turn, visual impairment and arthritis or neurological changes in the hands may compromise the self-administration of insulin.

Patients are particularly bad at adhering to dietary instructions, and the problem increases with age (Tunbridge and Wetherill 1970). Major barriers are that it requires a high degree of motivation to adhere to a reducing diet, and that the cultural, social and economic background of the patient may make the diet inappropriate (West 1973). Misconceptions as to the purpose of the diet and the theoretical basis of regimens and choices create further hurdles, particularly if the misconceptions are in the mind of the professional as well as the patient and relatives. One message which must be learnt by both patients and relatives, is the importance of patients on insulin or sulphonylurea drugs having regular meals and snacks. It should also be emphasised that a sudden increase in physical exertion, particularly in inactive individuals, may provoke hypoglycaemia. Patients should learn to anticipate this by taking extra carbohydrate.

The problem of older patients treating themselves with insulin was illustrated by the observations that older patients made more individual errors in the injection of insulin, and that, even if patients with impaired vision, co-ordination or mental function were excluded, the errors were considerably greater than these in younger patients (Kesson and Bailie 1981; Puxty et al. 1983).

Patients and relatives should be given specific education on the nature and management of diabetes mellitus. Recent experience suggests that this is deficient in all diabetics, but particularly the elderly, especially those with NIDDM (Knight et al. 1983). Aspects which should receive particular attention are insulin manipulation during illness and exercise; the theory and practice of a diabetic diet and carbohydrate exchange; the symptoms of hyper- and hypoglycaemia; and the complications of diabetes.

Education about diabetes is best conducted on a formal rather than an informal basis. Increasingly, diabetic day units or education centres are being developed, staffed by diabetes nurse specialists, and with dieticians and chiropodists available (Beggan et al. 1982). All new patients are instructed on a one-to-one basis or small group, and a manual is used to standardise information. Such centres may also provide a focus for continuing education of patients and serve as a point of contact when problems arise. Experience of formal education for elderly diabetics is limited, but there is evidence that there is a need for it and that patients would be receptive towards it (Knight et al. 1983). It is disappointing to note, however, that the correlation between the level of patient knowledge and laboratory markers of control is poor. Whether this is because patients who know how to control diabetes fail to implement the information, is not clear.

If an elderly patient on insulin has visual problems it may be useful to supply a preset syringe. It is more difficult to cope with the problem of reduced manual dexterity. If a relative is not available, regular visits from a district nurse should be arranged. In this situation there may have to be a compromise between close glycaemic control and the frequency of injections for which visits are practicable. If the problem is drawing up the insulin rather than the injection, then the district nurse or carer can draw up the evening injection at the same time as the morning injection and leave it in the refrigerator, ready for use by the patient himself at the appropriate time. There are no problems with this if a single preparation or a commercial pre-mixture is being used, and if the insulin is only going to be in contact with the syringe for less than 24 h. The introduction of pen injectors containing cartridges of premixed insulins (e.g. Noropen II) may facilitate self-administration of insulin by elderly subjects.

Monitoring Glycaemic Control

Accurate control of diabetes mellitus is dependent upon an effective and practicable system of monitoring blood glucose status. Traditionally, this has been done by measuring the urinary glucose concentration. There is, however, a wide inter-individual variation in the correlation between urine and blood glucose status

(Hayford et al. 1983). In old people there is the further problem that the renal threshold for glucose may be high so that negative urinalysis may accompany a blood glucose of 15 mmol/l. Control monitored by urine glucose levels is often poor. If this method is to be used, then a variety of methods are available. Of these the dipstick methods score in convenience over older methods using tablets, test tubes and water droppers. Double voiding regimens are unlikely to be complied with, or indeed to improve results materially.

If patients are able to cooperate, and the information obtained is likely to affect management they should be encouraged to monitor capillary blood glucose (Martin et al. 1986). Automated finger-pricking devices with visually read reagent strips are now widely used for insulin-dependent and increasingly for non-insulin-dependent subjects. Patients can use these provided they have no problems of manual dexterity or of vision. Automated reading of these strips by portable meters may be of value to the visually impaired. However, they require instruction in the development of a meticulous measurement technique. In achieving initial control, patients should perform tests relatively frequently, the timing of specimens depending on the insulin regimen being used. Once control has been stabilised, the frequency of testing by the patient or his carer can be reduced. Avoiding hypoglycaemia is the prime objective. This can often be achieved by performing a late-afternoon or late-evening test once a week. If more meticulous glycaemic control is necessary in a patient with a particular problem (e.g. painful neuropathy), then testing will need to be done more frequently, perhaps four pre-prandial tests per day or 2 days per week.

Once negative urinalysis is achieved in a patient taking oral hypoglycaemic agents he is likely to be symptom-free and he can be instructed to test his urine weekly, fasting or pre-prandially and 1–2 h after a main meal.

In a patient in whom it is considered desirable to achieve good glycaemic control then home blood glucose monitoring (fasting and 2 h post-prandially) should be considered and it may be necessary for a relative or carer to perform this. It should be remembered, however, that in the non-insulin-dependent diabetic there is an excellent correlation between the fasting blood glucose and overall glycaemic control, as assessed by the glycosylated haemoglobin, while a random post-prandial blood glucose also gives a satisfactory correlation with this (Paisey et al. 1980). It is, therefore, relatively easy for the general practitioner or clinic doctor, or indeed the district nurse or health visitor, to assess the efficacy of the patient's therapy on periodic estimations of blood glucose.

While the measurement of glycosylated haemoglobin has had a major impact on the management of younger patients with IDDM, this is probably not the case with older patients suffering primarily from NIDDM where, as noted above, the fasting blood glucose concentration is an excellent guide to glycaemic control. Nonetheless, the glycosylated haemoglobin may be of value in some elderly patients with NIDDM, perhaps identifying those patients who only make an effort to comply with therapy prior to clinic visits. Glycosylated haemoglobin remains a useful test in the elderly patient with IDDM, in whom an unexpectedly low value may point to periods of unsuspected mild hypoglycaemia.

It appears that in healthy subjects there is no effect of ageing on glycosylation of haemoglobin, nor indeed on other plasma proteins and albumin. While glycosylated haemoglobin assesses overall glycaemic control over the average lifespan of circulating red blood cells, plasma proteins are shorter-lived and glycosylation of them gives a shorter-term assessment of glycaemic control (1–2 weeks). These glycosylated proteins can now be simply, rapidly and cheaply assayed as fructosamine (Smart et al. 1988). However, the exact place of this assay in the management of diabetics in general and elderly patients in particular remains to be clarified.

It could be argued that old people have a limited life expectancy and that an attempt to prevent complications of diabetes by careful control is irrelevant. However, the mean life expectancies of men and women of 65 years are over 10 and 15 years respectively (Table 5.4) (Registrar General Scotland 1984). Reasonable control of diabetes during this period might therefore be expected to prolong life, and prevent some of the painful and incapacitating disorders which afflict elderly diabetics. The case cannot be made in extreme old age. Indeed, there is no evidence that, in patients over 75 years, NIDDM is associated with an excessive mortality (Parving 1987). Close control is also contraindicated in patients already severely afflicted by the complications of diabetes or coincidental pathology, such as severe dementia.

Table 5.4   Life expectancy of men and women in Scotland aged 65 years and over (Registrar General Scotland 1984).

Age (years)	Life expectancy (years)	
	Men	Women
65	12.5	16.5
75	7.6	10.2
85	4.5	5.6

Organisation of Care

Clearly this is dependent on local facilities. Every patient (and his relatives/carers) should have the opportunity of at least one consultation with a dietician. Ideally they should also receive some form of structured teaching about diabetes in a form appropriate to the patient. This may be at a GP mini-clinic or from a diabetes nurse specialist or health visitor. Patients should be regularly reviewed to supervise metabolic control, to review the need for medication, to search for particular problems and to screen for complications. In particular, regular inspection of the feet, measurement of blood pressure, checking of visual acuity and fundoscopy are important. There is evidence to suggest that patients can be as effectively followed up by GPs as by hospital clinics, provided that GP care is structured (e.g. in regular mini-clinics) and that the importance to patients of regular attendance for follow up is emphasised. Clearly, it may be more important for an infirm elderly diabetic to be visited regularly at home by his GP.

Detection of visual problems poses particular problems, particularly if a patient has cataract which may obscure the assessment of retinopathy. An additional problem is that few GPs are skilled at fundoscopy, although there is evidence that ophthalmic opticians can provide a useful (and at present free) screening service for significant diabetic eye disease. If there is any concern about the adequacy of visual follow-up, then the patient should attend either a specialist diabetic clinic or eye clinic on an annual basis at least.

Hospital diabetic clinics tend to concentrate on diabetes, while elderly patients may well be suffering from degenerative disease affecting multiple systems, the diabetes being the least of their problems. If specialist care of such patients is indicated then they may be better supervised in the geriatric clinic or day hospital, rather than a diabetic clinic.

Diabetic Coma

Ketoacidosis (Gill and Alberti 1985a)

The treatment of this condition is essentially the same in any age group though, in old age, a general impairment of homeostasis makes accurate calculation and monitoring of fluid, electrolyte and insulin replacement particularly critical (Schade and Eaton 1983). An elderly patient with DKA should ideally be observed in an intensive care unit. Central venous pressure monitoring may help to optimise fluid replacement, though management of this can be hazardous in a confused elderly patient. If the patient is drowsy or unconscious he should be given subcutaneous heparin 5000 units twice daily to lessen the risk of venous thrombosis. Table 5.5 summarises treatment (Gill and Alberti 1985a).

Table 5.5. Intravenous therapy in diabetic ketoacidosis

Insulin					
5–10 U/h until blood glucose <14 mmol/l and then, 3 U/h (add 50 g of glucose per litre of infusion here)					
Potassium					
20 mmol/h (modify depending on serum K+ level)					
Isotonic saline					
Hours of therapy	1	2	3	4	5+
Amount (litres)	1.5	1	1	1	0.5

Non-ketotic Hyperglycaemic Hyperosmolar Coma (Gill and Alberti 1985b)

The management of this is similar to that of DKA, but the emphasis should be on cautious rather than rapid correction of the metabolic disturbance (Fulop 1984). Since these patients are relatively sensitive to insulin, this should initially be infused at a rate of 5 U/h, and even this rate may need to be reduced. Hypotonic (N/2) saline should only be used if the serum sodium is greater than 145 mmol/l and should be changed for normal saline once the serum sodium returns to normal. Patients should always receive low dose heparin. Improvement of consciousness is usually slow and lags well behind the improvement in metabolic parameters. In the long term, diabetes in the majority of these patients can be controlled with diet alone, or diet plus oral hypoglycaemic agents.

Lactic Acidosis (Gill and Alberti 1985c)

Initial management of lactic acidosis in association with the use of biguanide drugs in diabetics aims firstly at rapid and total correction of the acidaemia by the infusion of large quantities (500–2000 mmol) of 2.7% sodium bicarbonate solution (150 mmol/500 ml), but care should be taken to avoid the sodium and fluid overload which this may entail. Central venous pressure monitoring is essential in the assessment of fluid balance in these patients who are often hypotensive. The efficacy of bicarbonate treatment is, however, unproven and indeed there is an argument that excessive bicarbonate replacement may be deleterious, by causing paradoxical worsening of intracellular acidosis (Ryder 1984). Other approaches include the use of a glucose potassium insulin infusion to stimulate pyruvate dehydrogenase activity. Haemo or peritoneal dialysis may be beneficial in severe cases and can be used not only to control fluid overload but also to correct acidaemia and remove any toxin (e.g. phenformin). Measures to correct hypotension by fluid and electrolyte and isotope administration may be necessary. A promising experimental approach is the use of dichloracetate. This enhances the activity of pyruvate dehydrogenase resulting in the conversion of lactate to pyruvate (Park and Arieff 1983). This agent improves survival in experimental animals and in man, but has not yet been evaluated in clinical trials.

Long-Term Complications

Prevention

There is now considerable circumstantial evidence that effective control of blood glucose concentrations reduces the incidence and severity of long-term complications. In patients with established retinopathy, this approach has produced an improvement in physiological tests of retinal function such as the oscillatory potential, and the macular recovery time (Lauritzen et al. 1983). It had no effect on the progression of morphological changes. This suggests that optimal treatment of diabetes may prevent the onset of retinopathy, but does not prevent progression of the disorder once vascular damage has been established. Since both retinal and renal damage are the result of similar microvascular changes, it might be expected that intensive management of diabetes would also prevent deterioration in renal function, and a recent study provided evidence for this (Fig. 5.1) (Holman et al. 1983). Since diabetic neuropathy may also be the result of microvascular damage, it is not surprising that the study also showed an improvement in vibration sense for patients on intensive treatment (Fig. 5.2).

An important caveat about these studies is that they relate to different forms of insulin therapy in insulin-dependent diabetes. Whether tighter control of blood glucose levels in older diabetics with NIDDM achieves similar benefits remains to be seen.

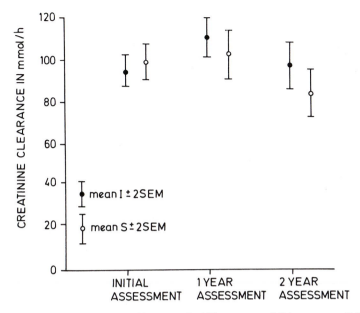

Fig. 5.1. Effects of intensive (I) and standard (S) treatment of diabetes on creatinine clearances. (After Holman et al. 1983.)

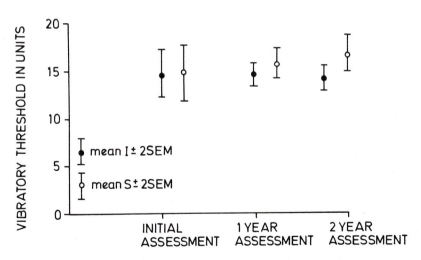

Fig. 5.2. Effects of intensive (I) and standard (S) treatment of diabetes on vibratory sensation thresholds. (After Holman et al. 1983.)

The effect of treatment of diabetes on large vessel disease is more contentious. Even if oral hypoglycaemic agents do not increase the risk of atherosclerosis there is no evidence that they decrease it (Jackson and Bressler 1981a, b). Intensive treatment with insulin reduces plasma levels of cholesterol and low density lipoprotein, but insufficient patient numbers have been studied to establish whether this diminishes the risk of cardiac, cerebral or peripheral vascular disease (Holman et al. 1983). It has indeed been suggested that hyperinsulinaemia is atherogenic (Stout 1987).

Treatment

Vision

Recent advances in ophthalmology including the use of artificial lens implants have greatly improved the quality of life of elderly patients with cataracts. Photo-coagulation techniques have also played a part in halting the rate at which vision deteriorates in patients with retinopathy (Herman et al. 1983). Since the major problem in elderly patients is diabetic maculopathy, it should be noted that treat-ment for this is more likely to be effective if the visual acuity is 6/12 or better at the time of photocoagulation treatment. This emphasises the previously mentioned role of regular screening of patients for diabetic eye disease by visual acuity testing as well as ophthalmoscopy. Recent advances in vitreous and intraocular surgery which have improved the management of advanced diabetic eye disease are unlikely to have wide applicability in elderly patients.

Renal Disease

In renal disease in younger patients with established diabetic nephropathy aggressive treatment of associated hypertension reduces the rate at which renal function deteriorates (Mogensen 1988). There is evidence that benefit can also be achieved in non-insulin-dependent patients. The pattern in the elderly patient, however, is more commonly that of hypertension in association with obesity and diabetes with no evidence of overt diabetic nephropathy. Control of hypertension in these circumstances has less effect on renal function. It is also important to remember that too vigorous an attack on hypertension may cause unacceptable side-effects (MacLennan et al. 1984).

Recurrent urinary tract infections lead to a deterioration in renal function and may lead to an acute complication such as renal papillary necrosis. The frequency of asymptomatic UTI in elderly diabetic females has already been commented on. Details of the principles underlying the management of urinary tract infections in the elderly are described elsewhere (Dontas 1984).

Diabetic Neuropathy

Painful diabetic neuropathy may occur in elderly patients and can be managed by a stepwise treatment protocol (Young and Clarke 1985). Initially simple analgesic and non-steroidal anti-inflammatory drugs are used and if these are ineffective, then the patient is started on an anti-depressant drug. Imipramine is the one most commonly used but may be substituted by mianserin in an elderly patient with cardiac disease. The effect is usually rapid but the dose may have to be increased to imipramine 150 mg/day or mianserin 90 mg at bed-time. In a recalcitrant case, the addition of a phenothiazine drug may be helpful, as may clonazepam if restless legs are a problem. In old age, it is particularly important to consider the dangers of toxicity from all these psychotropic agents. Uncontrolled observation in younger patients has shown that acute painful neuropathies may respond well to intensive insulin therapy and tight metabolic control. Anticonvulsant drugs such as carbamazepine and phenytoin have occasionally proved helpful, while drugs inhibiting aldose reductase are under evaluation.

Another common neurological problem in elderly patients is diabetic femoral neuropathy (amyotrophy). This is often painful and associated with weakness, weight loss (occasionally severe), and depression. It may be wrongly diagnosed as a terminal illness. In addition to measures directed towards the management of pain, insulin should be given to optimise glycaemic control. This usually also reverses weight loss and may help the neuropathy. The disorder is usually self-limiting but may take up to 2 years to resolve. Often insulin can be discontinued as the patient improves, and if glycaemic control can be maintained by other means.

Isolated cranial nerve palsies such as third nerve palsies require no specific treatment and usually resolve over 3 months or so. Peroneal nerve palsies causing foot drop require assessment in the Physiotherapy Department and may require an ankle splint.

The Diabetic Foot and Foot Ulceration

Foot problems in diabetics represent a major drain on health care resources. Elderly patients are most affected because age-related problems such as poor sight and arthritis make it difficult for them to see or touch their feet. Since the prevention of established foot lesions is critical it is important to ensure that the patients and their carers pay regular attention to their feet, and that they have regular attention from a chiropodist. Surveillance from other agencies including the district nurse, health visitor or general practitioner may also be necessary. Since most lesions develop following some form of trauma, often followed by infection, it is prevention which must be emphasised and it is here that the role of education is vital.

Established foot lesions in diabetics can be subdivided into those which are primarily ischaemic, and typical of the obese elderly non-insulin-dependent diabetic, and those which are primarily neuropathic and typical of the long-standing insulin-dependent diabetic.

Patients with primarily ischaemic lesions usually have distal (below knee) large vessel disease, but this may be complicated by a component of small vessel disease. They may first present with claudication, progress to rest pain in the foot and go on to suffer ulceration. This is usually painful and commonly involves either the heel, the great toe or the first (medial aspect) or fifth (lateral aspect) metatarsal head. The final stage is a painful gangrenous area and if this affects a toe it may be dry and mummified or infected and moist.

In such patients the circulation to the limb should be investigated, measuring systolic pressure gradients with a Doppler probe. In up to 10% of diabetic patients, however, systolic pressures are unreliable because of medial calcification of the posterior tibial artery.

Doppler studies point to the level of a blockage and if vascular reconstruction is contemplated, arteriography should be organised. Localised aorto-iliac disease or femoro-popliteal disease may be treated with reconstructive surgery (Reinhold, et al. 1979). Angioplasty of an isolated proximal stenosis is also effective and, by comparison, a relatively minor procedure. Distal reconstructions are technically more difficult and are still under evaluation.

Unfortunately, the majority of ischaemic foot lesions are not amenable to reconstruction and require conservative management. This includes avoidance of peripheral oedema appropriate cleansing and dressing, and antibiotic therapy depending on bacteriology results.

If the main problem is rest pain in the foot then chemical lumbar sympathectomy may be of value.

In an elderly patient, decisions on amputation are always worrying. If a toe has distal gangrene, careful management may permit mummification and autoamputation, avoiding the need for a surgical procedure. If there is persistent ischaemic ulceration elsewhere in the foot, or if rest pain is persistent, amputation is necessary. The problem remains of deciding on the level of amputation to provide a stump which will heal satisfactorily. Thermography may be helpful in this situation. Since the patient's peripheral vascular disease is usually a marker for co-existent coronary disease, his or her life expectancy may be limited and it may be kinder to amputate sooner rather than later. A below-knee amputation to relieve generalised pain may improve quality of life substantially, even if rehabilitation with an artificial limb is not realistic.

If the lesion is primarily neuropathic and sited typically under a metatarsal head, it is often painless and the foot warm with good pulses. The lesion is often at a pressure point and surrounded by callus.

A skilled chiropodist should remove the callus so that the floor of the ulcer is exposed. This allows the ulcer to drain and heal from its edges (Edmonds 1986). The ulcer should also be swabbed for bacteriological culture and appropriate antibiotics prescribed. It should be cleaned daily with a mild antiseptic and protected with a non-adhesive dressing.

If there is evidence of cellulitis, the patient should be admitted to hospital and given intravenous antibiotic therapy in the form of penicillin, flucloxacillin and metronidazole, pending the results of swab and blood cultures (Edmonds 1986). Attention should also be given to maintaining glycaemic control by insulin if necessary at this stage. Weight bearing must be prevented by bed rest and the ulcer regularly irrigated with sodium hypochlorite solution. The wound should be debrided and any abscess cavities drained. If digital gangrene or osteomyelitis of the underlying bone have developed, an amputation may be necessary (Edmonds 1986).

A reduction of weight-bearing forces is extremely important in neuropathic lesions. In an ambulant patient, lightweight plastercasts can be used to redistribute weight-bearing forces and allow healing of the ulcer (Burden et al. 1983). Once these lesions are healed, then recurrence should be prevented by redistributing weight-bearing forces with specialised footwear (Edmonds 1986).

The neuropathic or Charcot joint in the diabetic foot is uncommon as is neuropathic oedema. These problems have recently been reviewed (Edmonds 1986).

Infection

The treatment of infections in patients with diabetes is similar to that for any patient. It is important to recognise, however, that they are at increased risk of sustaining an infection and that once established it is likely to progress more rapidly. Apparently minor infections of the skin and subcutaneous tissues of the abdominal wall or perineum may be an early manifestation of extensive underlying necrotising fasciitis. It is important that such infections are identified early as they require aggressive surgical debridement of affected tissues and intensive antibiotic therapy. Measures aimed at the prevention and early identification of infections are therefore important. One of many examples is that elderly diabetics should have an annual injection with an appropriate influenza vaccine (Feely et al. 1983). This both produces an effective immunological response and does not have an adverse effect on carbohydrate metabolism.

References

Bailey CJ (1988) Metformin revisited: its actions and indication for use. Diabetic Medicine 5: 315–320

Beggan MP, Cregan D, Drury MI (1982) Assessment of the outcome of an education programme of diabetes self care. Diabetologia 23: 246–251

Berger W (1971) 88 Schwere Hypoglykamiezwischenfälle unter der Behandlung mit Sulfonylhamstoppen. Schweiz Med Wochenschr 71: 1013–1022

Burden AC, Jones GR, Jones R, Blandford RL (1983) Use of the "Scotchcast boot" in treating diabetic foot ulcers. Br Med J 286: 1555–1557

Campbell IW (1984) Metformin and glibenclamide: comparative risks. Br Med J 289: 289

Dandona P, Fonseca V, Mier A, Beckett AG (1983) Diarrhoea and metformin in a diabetic clinic. Diabetes Care 6: 472–474

Dontas AS (1984) Urinary tract infections and their implications. In: Brocklehurst JC (ed) Urology in the elderly. Churchill Livingstone, London, pp 162–192

Edmonds ME (1986) The diabetic foot. Pathophysiology and treatment. Clin Endocrinol Metab 15: 889–916

Feely BJ, Hartman LJ, Hampson AW, Proietto J (1984) Influenza immunisation in adults with diabetes mellitus. Diabetes Care 6: 475–478

Fuessel S, Adrian TE, Bacarese-Hamilton AJ, Bloom SR (1986) Guar in NIDD: effect of different modes of administration on plasma glucose and insulin responses to a starch meal. Practical Diabetes 3: 258–260

Fulop M (1984) The treatment of severely uncontrolled diabetes mellitus. Adv Intern Med 29: 327–353

Gill GV, Alberti KGMM (1985a) Management of diabetic ketoacidosis. Practical Diabetes 2: 115–120

Gill GV, Alberti KGMM (1985b) Hyperosmolar non-ketotic coma. Practical Diabetes 2: 20–35

Gill GV, Alberti KGMM (1985c) Lactic acidosis. Practical Diabetes 2: 15–19

Hayford JT, Weydert JA, Thompson RG (1983) Validity of urine glucose measurement for estimating plasma glucose concentrations. Diabetes Care 6: 40–44

Herman WH, Teutsch SM, Sepe SJ et al. (1983) An approach to the prevention of blindness in diabetes. Diabetes Care 6: 608–613

Holman RR, Mayon-White V, Orde-Peckar C et al. (1983) Prevention of deterioration of renal and sensory-nerve function by more intensive management of insulin dependent diabetic patients. Lancet 1: 204–208

Jackson JE, Bressler R (1981a) Clinical pharmacology of sulphonylurea hypoglycaemic agents: part 1. Drugs 22: 211–245

Jackson JE, Bressler R (1981b) Clinical pharmacology of sulphonylurea hypoglycaemic agents: part 2. Drugs 22: 295–320

Kesson CM, Bailie GR (1981) Do diabetic patients inject accurate doses of insulin? Diabetes Care 4: 333
Knight PV, Cummins AG, Kesson CM (1983) Elderly diabetics: a case for education. J Clin Exp Gerontol 5: 285–294
Kolterman OG (1987) The impact of sulphonylureas on hepatic glucose metabolism in type II diabetics. Diabetes Metab Rev 3: 399–414
Lauritzen T, Larson H, Frost-Larson K et al. (1983) Effect of 1 year of near-normal blood glucose levels on retinopathy in insulin-dependent diabetics. Lancet 1: 200–203
MacLennan WJ, Shepherd AN, Stevenson IH (1984) Treatment in clinical medicine: the elderly. Springer-Verlag, Berlin Heidelberg New York, pp 42–50
Martin BJ, Kesson CM (1986) Dietary control of elderly diabetic patients – a case for review. Practical Diabetes 3: 146–148
Martin BJ, Young RE, Kesson CM (1986) Home monitoring of blood glucose in elderly non-insulin dependent diabetics. Practical Diabetes 3: 37
Mogensen CE (1988) Management of diabetic renal involvement and disease. Lancet 1: 867–870
Mutch WJ, Dingwall-Fordyce I (1985) Is it a hypo? Knowledge of the symptoms of hypoglycaemia in elderly diabetic patients. Diabetic Medicine 2: 54–58
Nattrass M (1986) Treatment of type II diabetes. Br Med J 292: 1033–1034
Paisey RB, Bradshaw P, Hartog M (1980) Home blood glucose concentrations in maturity onset diabetes. Br Med J 280: 596–598
Parving G (1987) Mortality and survival in type 2 (non-insulin-dependent) diabetes mellitus. Diabetologia 30: 123–131
Park RT, Arieff AI (1983) Lactic acidosis: current concepts. Clin Endocrinol Metab 12: 339–358
Peden N, Newton RW, Feely J (1983) Oral hypoglycaemic agents. In: Feely J (ed) New drugs. British Medical Association, London, pp 106–113
Puxty JAH, Hunter DH, Burr WA (1983) Accuracy of insulin injection in elderly patients. Br Med J 287: 1762
Reaven GM (1985) Beneficial effect of moderate weight loss in older patients with NIDDM poorly controlled by insulin alone. J Am Geriatr Soc 33: 93–95
Registrar General Scotland (1984) Annual report. HMSO, London, p 94
Reinhold RB, Gibbons GW, Wheelock FC, Hoar CS (1979) Femoro-popliteal bypass in elderly diabetic patients. Am J Surg 137: 549–555
Ryder REJ (1984) Lactic acidosis: high dose or low dose bicarbonate therapy. Diabetes Care 7: 99–102
Schade DS, Eaton RP (1983) Diabetic ketoacidosis – pathogenesis, prevention and treatment. Clin Endocrinol Metab 12: 321–338
Shuman CR (1984) Optimum insulin use in older diabetics. Geriatrics 39 (October): 71–89
Smart LM, Howie AF, Young RJ et al. (1988) Comparison of fructosamine with glycosylated haemoglobin and plasma proteins as measures of glycaemic control. Diabetes Care 11: 433–436
Stout RW (1987) Insulin and atheroma: an update. Lancet 1: 1077–1079
Tattersall RB (1984) Diabetes in the elderly – a neglected area? Diabetologia 27: 167–173
Tattersall RB, Scott AR (1987) When to use insulin in the maturity onset diabetic. Postgrad Med J 63: 859–864
Teuscher A, Berger WG (1987) Hypoglycaemia unawareness in diabetics transferred from beef/porcine insulin to human insulin. Lancet 2: 382–385
Tunbridge R, Wetherill JH (1970) Reliability and cost of diabetic diets. Br Med J 2: 78–80
West K (1973) Diet therapy of diabetes: an analysis of failure. Ann Intern Med 79: 425–434
Wilson EA, Hadden DR, Merrett JD, Montgomery DAD, Weaver JA (1980) Dietary management of maturity onset diabetes. Br Med J 280: 1367–1369
Young RJ, Clarke BF (1985) Pain relief in diabetic neuropathy: the effectiveness of imipramine and related drugs. Diabetic Medicine 2: 363–366

6 Gonadal and Sexual Function

The effects of age and the menopause on pituitary and gonadal function in women have been discussed in Chap. 1. These affect not only sexual function, but a wide range of other physiological processes including resistance to infection, control of micturition, lipid metabolism, mood and bone formation (Sarles and Bremner 1982). Changes in men are less dramatic and more varied, but nonetheless important. A caveat is that hormonal function is just one of a wide range of factors which influence sexual behaviour in old age. Social attitudes, psychological expectations and physical health are equally if not more important.

Post-Menopausal Changes

The menopause is defined as being the last physiological menstrual period of a female, and in normal circumstances this is considered as having occurred if amenorrhoea has persisted for 12 months (Wallace et al. 1979). In developed countries the mean age for this is 50 years with a range between 42 and 58 years. While post-menopausal changes may continue into old age, the bulk of the published research concentrates on the years soon after the menopause.

Skin

Lack of oestrogen accelerates ageing changes in the skin. Amongst these are thinning of the epidermis, and a reduction in the amount of collagen and elastic tissue in the dermis. The number of sebaceous glands is reduced as is their secretion so that the skin becomes dry, itchy and less resistant to infection.

There is a diffuse loss of hair follicles in the scalp and surviving hairs are thin and brittle. Changes in facial, truncal, limb, axillary and pubic hair are dependent upon the relative concentrations of androgens and oestrogens. If the reduction in oestrogen secretion has exceeded that of androgens, elderly women may develop hirsutism. A parallel decline in both results in generalised hair loss.

Oestrogen replacement therapy delays skin and hair changes, but its potential side-effects are such that its use cannot be justified in this situation. A more appropriate approach is to encourage the patient to use an emulsifying ointment and lubricant bath oils. Monilial infections presenting as an intertrigo or vulvitis should be treated with an appropriate topical antifungal preparation such as nystatin ointment or miconazole cream.

Bone

Post-menopausal bone loss and its treatment are described in Chap. 7.

Cardiovascular Disorders

Seventy-five per cent of women experience vasomotor symptoms after the menopause. These are self-limiting and rarely persist for more than 4 years, so they do not present problems in the care of the elderly.

A more important issue is whether a reduction in oestrogen secretion increases the risk of cardiovascular and cerebrovascular disease. Certainly, after the menopause there is a rise in both serum cholesterol and serum very low density lipoprotein concentrations (Furman 1968). Evidence that this leads to disease is the finding that in post-menopausal women there was a higher incidence of coronary artery disease, congestive cardiac failure, stroke, and peripheral vascular disease than an age matched group of pre-menopausal subjects (Kannel et al. 1976). Evidence is accumulating that oestrogen replacement therapy protects against development of symptomatic coronary heart disease and certainly such therapy has beneficial effects on serum lipid profiles lowering LDL and increasing HDL (Judd 1987).

Urogenital Tract

After the menopause, the vaginal mucosa becomes thin, dry and atrophic. Histological changes include a reduction in the total thickness of the epithelium, associated with a reduction in the number of superficial cells, but an increasing quantity of basal cells. The practical relevance of these changes is that superficial cells have small deeply staining nuclei, whereas those of the basal cells are larger. Vaginal smears can therefore be used to assess the severity of postmenopausal changes and their response to treatment.

The elasticity of the vaginal wall is reduced (Masters and Johnson 1981). This combined with a reduction in lubrication means that sexual intercourse is more likely to result in mucosal fissuring. The resultant discomfort may precipitate vaginismus.

During orgasm the uterus may develop peristaltic contractions, but in old age these may be replaced by segmental contractions, similar to those associated with presbyoesophagus.

If the vaginal changes are troublesome they should be treated with topical oestrogens. These are available either as creams or pessaries and should be given for short courses of 1–2 weeks and then gradually withdrawn (Table 6.1). After treatment with oestrogens is completed, non-allergic moisturisers should be used to provide adequate lubrication before intercourse. Patients should also be advised that regular coitus may delay involutional changes.

Table 6.1. Commonly used topical oestrogen

Proprietary name	Generic preparation	Dose
Stilboestrol	500 µg stilboestrol	2 pessaries/night
Hormofemin	0.025% dienoestrol	½–1 applicatorful/daily
Ortho Dinoestrol	0.01% dienoestrol	1–2 applicatorful/daily
Ovestin	0.1% oestriol	1 applicatorful/daily
Premarin	625 µg/conjugated oestrogens	1–2 g daily (by calibrated applicator)

Note: This list merely gives examples and is not intended to be comprehensive.

Since the epithelium on the urethra and trigone has the same embryological derivation as the epithelium of the vagina, it also becomes atrophic after the menopause. Symptoms include frequency, dysuria and, in severe cases, urinary incontinence.

The condition can be treated with a 6-week course of an oral oestrogen, say, ethinyloestradiol, in a dose of 10–20 µg daily. Withdrawal is usually accompanied by endometrial haemorrhage. The synthetic oestrogen quinestradol does not have this effect. Its dose is 500 µg twice daily for 6 weeks. Topical preparations listed in Table 6.1 are also effective, but may be inappropriate if an old lady has mental and physical incapacity, and thus has difficulty in inserting the cream or pessary.

Endometrial Carcinoma

Despite the fact that reduced oestrogen levels decrease the risk of developing carcinoma of the body of the uterus, there is a steady rise in the death rate from endometrial carcinoma with increasing age (Registrar General Scotland 1984). There is the observation that women with obesity are at particular risk (Table 6.2) (Wynder et al. 1966). The correlation is thought to be due to the fact that adipose tissue converts androstenedione to oestrone, which is in turn converted to oestra-

Table 6.2. Relative risks of endometrial cancer related to height and weight (Wynder et al. 1966)

Weight	Height		
	<5'2"	5'2"–5'6"	>5'6"
> 10 lb below average	0.46	0.85	0.99
Average ± 9 lb	0.62	1.00	1.85
>10 lb above average	0.62	2.77	4.15

diol. By these mechanisms, obese postmenopausal women have higher circulating levels of oestrogens than do their non-obese counterparts.

Psychiatric Changes

An increase in the prevalence of anxiety, insomnia and depression is traditionally associated with the immediate post-menopausal period. However, while these symptoms are common in middle-aged women, they bear little relationship to the time of the menopause (McKinlay and Jeffreys 1974). Again, treatment of post-menopausal women with oestrogens has no more effect on psychological symptoms than a placebo (Thomson and Oswald 1977).

In old age, there is such a wide range of social, endocrine and neurobiochemical changes that it would be difficult to attribute an increase in the prevalence of depression to oestrogen deficiency (Blazer 1982).

Sexual Function

There are many misconceptions about sexual activity in old age (Felstein 1980). One is that it is closely linked to procreative ability and thus inevitably declines. This has in the past been reinforced by Western religious teaching which emphasises that procreation is the prime reason for sexual intercourse. The current view is that sexual activity is an integral part of a close relationship, particularly where this is linked with marriage and a family. In this situation there is no reason why changes in physiological function need determine behaviour.

There is also the misconception that physical attraction is inevitably associated with youth and beauty. In practice, conversation, mode of dress, range of mutual interests, personality and religious, educational and cultural backgrounds are equally important and less affected by ageing.

Emphasis has also been placed upon the importance of both general health and the condition of genital organs in maintaining a satisfactory sexual relationship. Obviously, old people with chronic ill health and severe physical incapacity are likely to have a restricted sexual life. However, even in extreme old age, only a minority of people have severe physical incapacity. It also requires re-emphasis that psychological factors are as important as physical ones in determining sexual satisfaction.

A number of studies have confirmed that the concept of there being a "cut-off" point to sexual activity is a myth. Level of interest and frequency of intercourse may decline but continues into old age (Gilmore 1973; Pfeiffer et al. 1972).

Although physical illness may interfere with sexual activity, careful investigation and imaginative treatment may minimise the problem (Felstein 1980). Patients with osteoarthritis may be instructed to take analgesics before intercourse, and advised on positioning. Again, treatment with L-dopa may reverse the loss of libido often associated with Parkinson's disease.

As in any age group, mental illness may affect sexual function. In elderly women the most common example is that depression reduces libido. This can often be reversed with appropriate antidepressant therapy. Increased sexual activity associated with organic brain disease is less of a problem in women than in men.

Social factors also influence sexual activity. An obvious example is that many elderly women have sexual inactivity imposed upon them by the death of their spouse. This is not a bar to other relationships, but younger people who may themselves have permissive attitudes to sex, often express abhorrence about similar relationships between two elderly lovers. This is no more apparent than in residential homes. Sexual segregation is no longer imposed, but any suggestion of intimacy between residents is often frowned upon. This may be justified if one of the partners has gross mental impairment, and is thus not capable of making rational decision. All too often it is indicative of ignorance and inadequate education of the staff.

Oestrogen Replacement

Clinical situations in which oestrogen therapy is of particular benefit are early post-menopausal vasomotor symptoms, genito-urinary atrophy and prevention of osteoporosis. However, the long-term effects of oestrogens remain uncertain, so long-term treatment can rarely be justified (Chap. 11). The most frequent indication for oestrogen therapy in elderly women is for atrophic changes in the urogenital tract as mentioned above, and in this situation, topical oestrogen therapy is normally prescribed. Whether the prescription of oral oestrogen replacement therapy in elderly women is ever indicated is unclear. Some elderly hysterectomised patients might prefer oral therapy to topical therapy, although in such patients, transdermal delivery of oestrogen is now an attractive alternative. The effect of oestrogen replacement therapy on prevention of bone loss may be limited

Table 6.3. Oestrogen and progestin calendar packs

1 Cyclo-Progynova 1 mg (Schering)	
Oestradiol valerate	1 mg daily for 11 days
Levonorgestrel	250 µg daily for 10 days
No treatment	7 days
2 Menophase (Syntex)	
Mestranol	12.5 µg daily for 5 days
Mestranol	25 µg daily for 8 days
Mestranol	50 µg daily for 2 days
Mestranol Norethisterone	25 µg 1 mg } daily for 3 days
Mestranol Norethisterone	30 µg 1.5 mg } daily for 6 days
Mestranol Norethisterone	20 µg 750 µg } daily for 4 days
3 Prempak 0.625 (Ayerst)	
Conjugated oestrogens	625 µg daily for 21 days
Norgesterel	500 µg daily for 7 days

Note: This list only provides examples and is not comprehensive.

to the first 10 years or so after the menopause, and thus the beneficial effects of such therapy in elderly women who have already suffered osteoporotic factors remain to be demonstrated.

If oestrogen therapy is to be prescribed, it is essential that the smallest effective dose should be used (Judd et al. 1981). It is also important that treatment should be discontinuous, so that the patient is only taking oestrogen 3 out of 4 weeks. Finally, the risk of endometrial hyperplasia and cancer is further reduced if a progestin is given concurrently. A variety of oestrogen and progestin preparations are available as calendar packs (Table 6.3). For previously hysterectomised women preparations allowing transdermal administration of oestrogen are now available. The apparent advantage of this delivery system is that active oestrogen is delivered into the systemic circulation where oestrogen is normally secreted, and not directly via the portal circulation to hepatocytes, which may be responsible for undesirable changes in renin substrate (leading to hypertension), in clotting factors (leading to thromboembolic phenomena) and in hepatic lipid metabolism (increasing cholesterol saturation of bile).

Women taking oestrogen should be reviewed at least annually when the blood pressure should be checked, and cardiovascular, breast and pelvic examination performed.

Elderly Men

The effects of ageing on testosterone secretion are gradual. This accounts in part for the fact that age changes in gonadal function in men produce few of the dramatic anatomical and physiological manifestations of this found in women. A statistical association between plasma testosterone levels and sexual activity has been reported in a group of very healthy elderly men (Tsitouras et al. 1982) but other factors such as physical and mental health and alcohol and tobacco intake have a far more important effect on potency (Davidson et al. 1983). Others found no correlation between free testosterone concentrations and indices of libido and sexual performance in ageing males and indeed found a positive correlation between plasma LH and performance (Davidson et al. 1982). In this study, age had an independent effect on both libido and sexual performance, but ageing affected libido less than potency.

Whatever the explanation, ageing is associated with a variety of changes in male sexual function (Masters and Johnson 1981). The first is that stimulation takes longer to produce complete penile engorgement, and that direct physical rather than indirect emotional stimulation becomes more and more important. Changes in gonadal and prostatic function mean that the force and volume of seminal fluid ejaculation is reduced. Accompanying this there is a reduction in the desire to ejaculate.

A consequence of these age changes is a reduction in the frequency of sexual intercourse (Pfeiffer et al. 1972). There also is a declining interest in sexual activity, though the decline is not as striking as that found in women. Though there is wide individual variation, there is no evidence that ageing is associated with an increase in atypical behaviour such as homosexuality (Felstein 1980).

Many ageing males fear impotence. Anxiety about its traditional association with old age may be sufficient to precipitate the condition. This can often be remedied by appropriate reassurance, after physical examination has excluded other problems.

The most important physical cause of impotence in old men is peripheral vascular disease. Another classic but less common cause is diabetic autonomic neuropathy. Common neurological disorders associated with impotence are cerebrovascular disease and Parkinsonism.

A wide range of drugs often used in old age may cause impotence. These include the tricyclic antidepressants, non-steroidal anti-inflammatory agents, beta-adrenoceptor-blocking agents, thiazide diuretics and cimetidine (Dukes 1984). Clear-cut hypogonadism is rarely the cause of impotence in the elderly (Davis et al. 1985).

Mental disorders may affect sexual activity. Examples are that both depression and anxiety may reduce libido or cause impotence. At the opposite extreme, organic brain disease may result in inappropriate sexual behaviour (Szasz 1983). In institutions this is often directed towards staff. The inappropriate behaviour may be verbal and consist of using foul language, describing past sexual activity, or suggesting a sex encounter. Physical acts include showing genitalia, touching or grabbing staff, undressing publicly, or masturbating publicly.

Staff often experience considerable difficulty in coping with such incidents or discussing these with their colleagues. There is advantage in discussing the problem during nursing education, and having staff meetings at which policies towards such incidents can be developed. More experienced staff develop strategies for dealing with episodes, and should be encouraged to counsel their more junior colleagues. It may be that the abnormal behaviour may be a manifestation of agitation or confusion, in which case the judicious use of a tranquilliser may be helpful. A more controversial approach is to attempt hormonal suppression of the overactivity. Cyproterone acetate in a dose of 50 mg twice daily can be used for this purpose. There have been no studies on the efficacy of the agent in this situation, but the possible association between androgen levels and sexual activity in elderly men suggests that it might have some benefit. Most clinicians have reservations about modifying behaviour in this way, and are only likely to use hormonal therapy as a last resort.

Androgen Replacement

The enthusiasm with which at the turn of the century doctors attempted to rejuvenate elderly men with testicular extracts has been largely discontinued. Nonetheless, there remain some authors who claim that treatment with an androgen increases sexual responsiveness in a large proportion of elderly men (Greenblatt et al. 1976). In a double-blind placebo-controlled experiment in elderly males with low normal testosterone levels, testosterone treatment was associated with improvement in erectile capacity measured by nocturnal penile tumescence and also by some improvement in sexuality. However, none of the measured parameters was restored to normal (Davidson et al. 1982). Further studies are required to establish these claims. Even if androgens are effective, certain of the synthetic androgens have serious side-effects which may well outweigh any benefit in terms of sexual performance (Chap. 11).

References

Blazer DG (1982) Depression in later life. Mosby, St Louis, pp 49–66

Davidson JM, Kwan M, Greenleaf WJ (1982) Hormonal replacement and sexuality in men. Clin Endocrinol Metab 11: 599–624

Davidson JM, Chen JJ, Crapo L et al. (1983) Hormonal changes and sexual function in ageing men. J Clin Endocrinol Metab 57: 71–77

Davis SS, Viosca SP, Guralnik M et al. (1985) Evaluation of impotence in older men. West J Med 142: 499–505

Dukes MNG (1984) Meyler's side effects of drugs. Elsevier, Amsterdam

Felstein I (1980) Sexual function in the elderly. Clin Obstet Gynecol 7: 401–420

Furman RH (1968) Are gonadal hormones of significance in the development of ischaemic heart disease? Ann NY Acad Sci 149: 922–933

Gilmore A (1973) Attitudes of the elderly to marriage. Gerontol Clin 15: 124–132

Greenblatt RB, Witherington R, Sipahioglu IB (1976) Hormones in sexual dysfunction. Drug Therapy 6: 101–104

Judd HL (1987) Oestrogen replacement therapy. Clin Endocrinol Metab 1: 177–206

Judd HL, Cleary RE, Creasman WT et al. (1981) Oestrogen replacement therapy. Obstet Gynecol 58: 267–275

Kannel WB, Hjortland MC, MacNamara PM (1976) Menopause and risk of cardiovascular disease; the Framingham study. Ann Intern Med 85: 447–452

Masters WH, Johnson VE (1981) Sex and the ageing process. J Am Geriatr Soc 29: 385–390

McKinlay SM, Jeffreys M (1974) The menopausal syndrome. Br J Prev Soc Med 28: 108–115

Pfeiffer E, Venvoerdt A, Davis GC (1972) Sexual behaviour in middle life. Am J Psychiatry 128: 1262–1267

Registrar General Scotland (1984) Annual report, HMSO, London

Sarles MR, Bremner WJ (1982) The menopause and climacteric: endocrinologic basis and associated symptomatology. J Am Geriatr Soc 30: 547–561

Szasz G (1983) Sexual incidents in an extended care unit for aged men. J Am Geriatr Soc 31: 407–411

Thomson J, Oswald I (1977) Effect of oestrogen on the sleep, mood and anxiety of menopausal women. Br Med J 2: 1317–1319

Tsitouras P, Martin CE, Harman SM (1982) Relationship of serum testosterone to sexual activity in healthy elderly men. J Gerontol 37: 288–293

Wallace RB, Sherman BM, Bean JA et al. (1979) Probability of menopause with increasing duration of amenorrhoea in middle-aged women. Am J Obstet Gynecol 135: 1021–1024

Wynder EL, Escher GC, Mantel N (1966) An epidemiological investigation of cancer of the endometrium. Cancer 19: 489–520

7 Bone Disease and Disorders of Calcium Homeostasis

A review of bone disease in the elderly would be inappropriate in this book. However, hormonal changes which are associated with ageing and the diseases of old age have a profound effect on bone metabolism, and it is this relationship which will be emphasised here.

Osteoporosis

Aetiology

Although there is a decline of bone mass in both men and women after the age of 35 years, the decline is most striking in women over the age of 50 years (Exton-Smith et al. 1969). The fact that an identical decline occurs in bone mass after oophorectomy suggests that hormonal changes associated with the menopause have an important effect on calcium metabolism.

The currently favoured hypothesis is that reduced oestrogen secretion renders bone more sensitive to the effects of parathyroid hormone (PTH), so that there is an increase in the resorption of calcium from bone (Paterson and MacLennan 1984). The resulting increase in the plasma calcium concentration has two consequences. Firstly, there is feedback inhibition of PTH secretion from the parathyroid glands, so that there is a reduction of the pressure on the small bowel to absorb dietary calcium. Secondly, an increased quantity of calcium is excreted in the urine. In combination, the effect of these two changes is to push post-menopausal women into negative calcium balance. If mild but persistent, this leads to bone rarefaction rather than skeletal decalcification.

In men the explanation for the progressive, though less striking, loss of bone mass with increasing age is less clear. Changes in the renal synthesis of 1,25-dihydroxyvitamin D (calcitriol), or in gonadal function may be factors, but their association with osteoporosis has been largely unexplained.

Though most old people have a reasonable intake of calcium, changes in its absorption and excretion mean that there is an increase in requirements, particularly in elderly women (Heaney et al. 1982). There is also evidence that the intake of calcium in earlier life may have an important influence on bone mass. An example is that, in Yugoslavia, the bone mass of people living in an area with a high calcium intake was higher than for individuals from an area in which this was low (Matkovic et al. 1979). Since old people who had a low maximum bone mass at maturity are more likely to develop osteoporosis this would appear to be a lifelong effect. In particular, a high calcium intake in youth is likely to produce a high bone mass at maturity, so that the risk of the individual having severe skeletal rarefaction in old age is reduced.

There also is an association between chronic renal failure and bone rarefaction (Feest et al. 1977). The basis for this is that the ability of the kidneys to convert 25-hydroxycholecalciferol (calcidiol) into the metabolically active 1,25-dihydroxycholecalciferol (calcidiol) is impaired. As a consequence there is a reduction in the gastro-intestinal absorption of calcium. The resultant hypocalcaemia stimulates the parathyroid gland to produce more PTH, and this causes bone resorption. Since there is a decline in both renal function and calcium absorption in old age, it is tempting to link the two together as a cause of the decline in bone mass associated with old age (Heaney et al. 1982). Certainly, serum calcitriol levels are often reduced in old age, but there is a considerable overlap in values for different age groups, so that the link has not yet been firmly substantiated.

Treatment with corticosteroids has an effect on bone metabolism, but has a particularly critical effect in old age where there often is a considerable degree of osteoporosis under baseline conditions. They exert this effect by suppressing the synthesis of collagen by osteoblasts and by stimulating the activity of osteoclasts (Jowsey and Riggs 1970). Corticosteroid excess also causes a reduction in the gastro-intestinal absorption of calcium, but the pathogenesis of this is unclear (Findling et al. 1982). While the severity of bone loss is related to the duration of treatment, there is no clear relationship with dosage (Hahn 1978). Thus, even small doses of corticosteroids put elderly patients at risk of osteoporosis and its complications. The only safe policy is to avoid corticosteroid therapy altogether in other than serious conditions such as giant cell arteritis and polymyalgia rheumatica.

Other endocrine disorders exacerbate bone rarefaction. An example is that hyperthyroidism produces an excess of osteoclastic activity (Jowsey and Deterbeck 1969). This is associated with an increased risk of fractures, particularly in women over the age of 50 (Fraser et al. 1971). Maturity onset diabetes also is associated with a reduced bone mass (Levin et al. 1976). The effect is marginal, however, and elderly diabetics do not have an increased incidence of fractured vertebrae or long bones (Heath et al. 1980). Primary hyperparathyroidism may also contribute to osteoporosis.

Clinical Features and Investigation

Osteoporosis causes a wedge-shaped collapse of the vertebral bodies resulting in back pain and the striking kyphosis seen in many elderly patients. A more serious consequence is an increase in the incidence of fractures of the lower radius in women between the ages of 50 and 60 years, and of the proximal femur and pelvis in women over 70 (Knoweldon et al. 1964).

A chest X-ray shows increased radiolucency and cortical thinning of the ribs, clavicles and humeri, while lateral views of the dorsal and lumbar regions reveal radiolucency and wedging of the vertebral bodies. Serum calcium, phosphate and alkaline phosphatase levels are usually within normal limits, but the latter may be elevated immediately after a fracture.

In investigational and intervention studies, assessment of bone mass is important and a number of methods are available for this. Single photon osteodensitometry is the most simple method and is applicable primarily to the radius, giving an index of cortical bone mass. Dual photon osteodensitometry is applicable to lumbar vertebrae. Computerised tomography is somewhat unwieldy but nonetheless is a very sensitive method for determining bone density and can be applied to vertebral bodies which consist predominantly of trabecular bone.

Prevention

Post-menopausal bone loss can be reduced by oestrogen replacement (Stevenson and Whitehead 1982). The risks of long-term side-effects are minimised by giving a low dose of oestrogen, by giving it cyclically in patients with a uterus, and by introducing a progesterone in the latter stages of each cycle (Chap. 6). Even with this approach, uncertainty of long-term effects is such that treatment should not be continued for more than 5 years.

Calcium supplements also reduce the rate of bone loss in post-menopausal women although the effect seems limited to compact rather than trabecular bone (Rhis et al. 1987), and, if given along with an oestrogen, they complement the effect of the latter (Nordin et al. 1980). A reasonable dose is calcium gluconate 1–2 g daily. Though this treatment is safe and can be continued indefinitely, the problem remains of identifying women at particular risk from osteoporosis. There is epidemiological evidence that women with bone densities in the lower tertiles of bone density in middle age are most likely to develop osteoporosis in old age, but there is a great deal of individual variation, so a radiological evaluation would lack specificity (Adams et al. 1970). Even if this were not the case, the routine radiological assessment of all middle-aged women would be costly and impracticable.

A particular situation in which calcium supplements are indicated is that of patients recently taken off an oestrogen. This may be followed by rapid bone loss unless there are adequate supplies of the mineral (Christiansen 1982). There may also be a place for the use of calcium supplements in elderly patients on corticosteroids, but their benefit in this situation has not yet been established.

While studies using vitamin D and its metabolites in the treatment of osteoporosis have not been encouraging there is evidence that supplementation with supra-physiological doses of vitamin D (15 000 iu of vitamin D weekly) for 2 years prevents loss of cortical bone in elderly women (Nordin et al. 1985).

Treatment

Since most agents prevent rather than reverse bone loss, they are of little value once the clinical features of osteoporosis have become apparent. This means that there is little place for the use of substances with potentially serious side-effects (such as the oestrogens) if a patient over 65 presents with symptoms related to osteoporosis. Calcium supplements have the marginal advantage of preventing further bone loss and do no harm, unless the patient suffers from nephrolithiasis. A simple preparation such as calcium gluconate is usually adequate in a minimum dose of 1.2 g daily. The mineral is also available as the bovine bone extract, microcrystalline hydroxyapatite compound (MCHC). Though this reduces bone loss, there is little evidence that it is more effective than other less expensive preparations.

Preliminary studies suggest that the oral anabolic steroid, stanozolol, may not only prevent bone rarefaction, but may actually increase bone mass (Chestnut et al. 1983). Balanced against this potential benefit is the worry that the drug may be hepatotoxic and affect plasma lipid concentrations, so that there may be a long-term increased risk of ischaemic heart disease (Taggart et al. 1982). Further evaluation is necessary, therefore, before stanazolol is used in the routine management of osteoporosis.

Vitamin D and its derivatives, calcitriol and alfacalcidol have been investigated in the management of osteoporosis. All increase calcium absorption but none reduces bone loss (Nordin et al. 1980; Chistiansen et al. 1981). Indeed, without calcium supplements, vitamin D may actually increase bone loss. Another hormone with a possible role in the treatment of osteoporosis is calcitonin. This not only suppresses osteoclastic activity but also stimulates that of osteoblasts (Mazzoli et al. 1986). Trials of its effect on bone mass have been promising. Major disadvantages are that it is expensive, and that it has to be given by injection over a prolonged period.

The osteosclerotic effects of fluoride have also been explored in the management of osteoporosis (Riggs et al. 1982). However, although bone formation is stimulated, the new bone is woven and poorly calcified and more susceptible to fracture. This has led to the concurrent use of calcium and vitamin D with fluoride, but, although large scale investigations are in progress, this combination is not yet of proven efficacy. Disadvantages are that the regimen is complex, and that radiographs give a misleading impression of the effect of the treatment on bone structure. Sodium fluoride is likely to prove more useful in the management of spinal rather than peripheral osteoporosis.

Osteomalacia

Aetiology

Vitamin D deficiency is a common concomitant of ill health and disability in old age (MacLennan 1979). It is a particular feature of men and women who have restricted mobility or are housebound (MacLennan et al. 1979). The critical factor here is that these two groups have an inadequate exposure to sunlight and ultraviolet irradiation. Without this, there is inadequate biosynthesis of cholecalciferol from cutaneous 7-dehydrocholesterol (Parfitt et al. 1982). Vitamin D can also be obtained from dietary sources, but the mean daily intakes of this for old people living at home range between 1.25 and 2.5 μg, figures comparing unfavourably with the minimum daily intakes of 2.5 μg recommended by the World Health Organisation (Omdahl et al. 1982). Sick old people thus have an inadequate exposure to sunlight and consume inadequate quantities of vitamin D to compensate for this. Previous gastric surgery and particularly partial gastrectomy further predispose to vitamin D deficiency and osteomalacia. Certain hepatic microsomal enzyme inducing drugs result in the metabolism and inactivation of vitamin D and cause hypocalcaemia and osteomalacia. The long-term use of phenytoin is an example.

Clinical Feature and Implications

Bone pain is common in the arms and legs, and is sometimes of such severity that the mistaken diagnosis of polymyalgia rheumatica is made. Though kyphosis and other skeletal deformities may be the result of osteomalacia, they are more usually the result of osteoporosis (Wigzell et al. 1981).

X-rays of the chest and pelvis show increased radiolucency and cortical thinning. In a proportion of patients, there also is the characteristic appearance of a pseudofracture (Looser's zone), a line of decalcification only partially traversing the width of a bone. As a diagnostic feature, this has high specificity, but low sensitivity.

The biochemical features of osteomalacia are those of low serum calcium and phosphate concentrations and an elevated alkaline phosphatase concentration, either alone or in combination. Although cases of osteomalacia with normal serum calcidiol levels have been reported, these are rare. If a patient with abnormal serum calcium, phosphate or alkaline phosphatase levels has a normal serum calcidiol level, a bone biopsy may be necessary to make a firm diagnosis. Alternatively, if the serum calcium, phosphate or alkaline phosphatase levels are abnormal and the serum calcidiol level low it is reasonable to assume that the patient has osteomalacia. Most patients with normal calcium, phosphate and alkaline phosphatase levels and a low calcidiol level do not have osteomalacia (Hodkinson and Hodkinson 1980). This means that, on its own, the serum calcidiol level is not a useful screening test for the disorder.

If a bone biopsy is performed, it shows that there is a normal quantity of bone, but that there is an increase in the amount of osteoid. The latter can be quantified by relating the volume of osteoid to total bone volume, by enumerating the percentage of surfaces covered by osteoid or by using polarised light to count the numbers of osteoid lamellae (Hodkinson and Hodkinson 1981).

Complications

One of the most common, but most frequently missed of these is a proximal myopathy, presenting as quadriceps wasting, weakness and tenderness associated with a waddling gait and inability to rise out of a chair (Schott and Wills 1976). The condition is often wrongly attributed to osteoarthritis of the hips, and, if there is severe tenderness, polymyalgia may be suspected. Though the myopathy is probably directly related to low concentrations of both calcidiol and calcitriol, its exact pathogenesis has not been elucidated (Kanis et al. 1982).

The importance of vitamin D deficiency as a cause of fractures of the proximal femur is uncertain (Parfitt et al. 1982). Many patients with fractures have histological evidence of osteomalacia, and low plasma calcidiol levels are more common in this group. This does not mean that the relationship is one of cause and effect. Many patients with fractured femurs suffer from conditions associated with ataxia and limited mobility, and these may cause both falls and inadequate exposure to sunlight (Cook et al. 1982).

Prevention

Apart from the small number of elderly patients with malabsorption, the only group at substantial risk of osteomalacia are those with restricted mobility. A reasonable policy might be to offer vitamin D supplements to housebound women over the age of 75 years. A daily table of calcium and vitamin D (BPC) containing 500 units of ergocalciferol is effective and safe (MacLennan and Hamilton 1977). It is important to ensure long-term compliance, however, and an alternative is to give a large single oral or parenteral dose of say 300 000 units of calciferol (Burns et al. 1985). One dose produces sustained elevation of plasma levels of calcidiol for at least 6 months, without significant risk of hypercalcaemia. Twice-yearly doses of 100 000 units calciferol orally has also been shown to be effective and safer (Davies et al. 1985).

Ingenious methods have also been devised for exposing long-stay residents and patients to ultra-violet irradiators installed as part of the lighting systems of a day area (Devgun et al. 1980). Such experiments have not been universally successful, and present the risk of causing long-term visual damage.

Treatment

The simplest form of treatment is to give a single oral or parenteral dose of 600 000 units of calciferol (Burns and Paterson 1985).

Since the dietary calcium intake may be low, calcium supplements should also be given as calcium gluconate 1200 mg daily in divided doses. Following this, the response of the serum calcium concentration should be measured at regular intervals. A single large dose of calciferol is usually sufficient to maintain serum calcium levels within normal limits for at least 6 months. Thereafter, the oral dose or injection should be repeated. The serum alkaline phosphatase concentration is an unreliable guide to the efficacy of treatment, since it may take anything up to a year to return to normal.

Though treatment produces a rapid improvement in bone pain and radiological abnormalities, its effect on impaired mobility and ability to transfer is less obvious

(Corless et al. 1985). This is because most old people with osteomalacia suffer from multiple pathology, and a proximal myopathy is just one of a wide range of reasons for them being unable to walk.

Hypercalcaemia

The advent of multichannel analysis of blood samples including the routine assessment of serum calcium has led to the identification of large numbers of elderly patients with hypercalcaemia. In the absence of associated symptoms and signs, this is often of little clinical significance, but because it may be indicative of serious underlying pathology it requires further investigations.

Primary Hyperparathyroidism

This is primarily a disease of old age, its prevalence rising from around 1 per 1000 of the population under 60 years, to one of 9 per 1000 over this age (Paterson and MacLennan 1984). Age also affects the presentation of the disease. Whereas peptic ulcers and renal calculi are common in young patients, these are rare in the elderly, many of whom are only identified during a routine estimation of their serum calcium level (Table 7.1). Old people also rarely present with skeletal radiological abnormalities or with fractures. They more often suffer from malaise, mental impairment, depression, tiredness or generalised weakness, but these are often mistakenly attributed to old age. It may only be after treatment of the hypercalcaemia that their relevance becomes apparent (Heath et al. 1980).

Table 7.1. Presentation of hyperparathyroidism in patients of different ages (Paterson and MacLennan 1984)

Presenting feature	Ages of patients (years)		
	0–49	50–69	70–99
Renal calculi	32%	12%	0%
Peptic ulcer	27%	3%	3%
Other clinical features	32%	33%	29%
Coincidental hypercalcaemia	9%	52%	68%
Total number	44	67	59

Eighty per cent of old people with hyperparathyroidism have a solitary adenoma, with 17% having generalised parathyroid hyperplasia, and only 3% having a carcinoma (Aldinger et al. 1982; Tibblin et al. 1983).

The most characteristic biochemical finding in elderly patients is hypercalcaemia, but the serum calcium level may be within normal intervals if a blood sample is taken during an acute intermittent illness such as a bronchopneumonia, urinary tract infection, myocardial infarction or pulmonary embolism. A particular problem in old age is that coincidental vitamin D deficiency may mask the biochemical effects of hyperparathyroidism (Stanbury 1981). The serum phosphate concentration is either low or a low normal, and, though the serum alkaline phosphate may be elevated, it is more usually normal. In interpreting serum calcium concentrations in elderly patients it is particularly important to make a correction for reduced serum protein levels. For example, a correction factor of 0.02 mmol/l is added to or subtracted from the measured serum calcium concentration for each 1 g/l which the serum albumin concentration lies below or above 40 g/l.

A wide range of tests has been used in the diagnosis of hyperparathyroidism. These include measurements of the tubular reabsorption of phosphate and urinary excretion of calcium and hydroxyproline. Corticosteroids (hydrocortisone 40 mg three times daily) do not suppress serum calcium in primary hyperparathyroidism, but do so in a proportion of cases in which hypercalcaemia is due to other causes. Nonetheless, all these tests have a low specificity, and have largely been replaced by assays of the serum parathyroid hormone (PTH) concentration (Boyd and Ladenson 1984). It is important to realise that some patients with primary hyperparathyroidism have PTH concentrations in the normal range, though this is inappropriately high for the prevailing serum calcium concentration. It is also important to remember that many commercial PTH assays measure variable amounts of inactive PTH fragments and this can on occasion make interpretation of results difficult (Hackeng et al. 1986).

Bone X-rays are of limited value in old people because the specific radiological features of hyperparathyroidism are either absent or masked by coincidental osteoporosis. An isotopic bone scan after the administration of technetium-99m bisphosphonate is more useful, in that there is a generalised increase in the uptake of the isotope. There are other skeletal disorders which produce a similar appearance, so that the test is not a substitute for performing a serum PTH assay.

If the hypercalcaemia associated with hyperparathyroidism is mild (<2.75 mmol/l) and is not associated with symptoms, then the patient may be left untreated and the clinical and biochemical status monitored at regular intervals (Heath et al. 1980; Paterson et al. 1984). In a study reported from Sweden untreated patients with mild hypercalcaemia had a better survival rate than normocalcaemic controls, but survival rates were similar in patients aged over 70 years (Palmer et al. 1987). It should be emphasised, however, that in an elderly patient with hyperparathyroidism, symptoms may be vague and non-specific, and that it is only after treatment that the patient realises how unwell he has felt. Clinical evaluation thus has to be skilled and painstaking.

If treatment is necessary, the treatment of choice is surgical removal of the offending gland. Age alone is no barrier to surgery (Heath et al. 1980). The only contra-indications are coincidental disease presenting an unacceptably high operative risk, or severe mental or physical incapacity unlikely to be resolved by parathyroidectomy. Most surgeons with experience in parathyroid surgery have a high success rate (90%) in locating a parathyroid adenoma at neck exploration. Hence pre-operative adenoma localisation procedures are not routinely indicated. However, where there has been previous surgery or recurrence of hyperparathyroidism after previous surgery, or where it is felt that a particularly short operation time is essential, then preoperative localisation procedures should be performed. Larger adenomas may be detected by ultrasound or CT scanning, while smaller ones may be identified using a double isotope procedure in which thallium-201 shows up thyroid and parathyroid tissues and technetium-99m identifies the thyroid gland, so that computer subtraction can be used to identify the parathyroid gland (Krubsack et al. 1986). Venous sampling for PTH concentrations in the neck veins with a catheter introduced via a femoral vein is a highly specialised technique, but may be useful in difficult cases.

Post-operatively, the patient may have mild problems with hypocalcaemia for up to 2 weeks. If this is asymptomatic then oral calcium supplements (1800 mmol/day) may be given. If this is inadequate, the patient should be started on 1 alpha hydroxyvitamin D_3 (alphacalcidol). Symptomatic hypocalcaemia with tetany requires immediate treatment with intravenous calcium gluconate. It is well recognised that patients with more severe hyperparathyroidism having higher serum calcium levels and significant osteitis fibrosa are particularly likely to have post-operative problems, presumably as calcium and phosphate are drawn into bone after removal of the PTH stimulus. In some patients hypomagnesaemia may compound the problem.

If patients are considered unfit or are unwilling to consent to surgery, medical treatment should be instituted. They should be encouraged to take plenty of oral fluids and oral phosphate therapy should be considered. Long-term treatment with phosphate causes extra-skeletal calcification with problems such as renal calculous disease and sometimes renal failure. The substance is also often poorly tolerated and causes diarrhoea. Sodium cellulose phosphate 5 g three times daily is usually used.

Hypercalcaemia and Malignancy

Hypercalcaemia and malignancy are usually associated with advanced disease. The commonly associated neoplasms are carcinoma of breast and bronchus and myeloma. Other causes are carcinoma of oesophagus, thyroid, prostate, kidney and bile ducts and lymphoproliferative disorders. Hypercalcaemia in malignancy is either the result of extensive osteoclastic activity associated with direct invasion of bone by tumour, or by tumour cells secreting humoral factors with osteoclastic activity. The nature of the pathology varies and has not been fully elucidated (Munday and Martin 1982). A number of substances have been implicated in the stimulation of bone resorption. These include prostaglandins, various growth factors and lymphokines. Lymphoproliferative tumours may produce calcitriol and other active sterols.

Recent work, however, has emphasised the similarities between humorally mediated hypercalcaemia of malignancy (HHM) and primary hyperparathyroidism. A number of groups of workers have now identified peptides secreted by tumours which appear to be responsible for the hypercalcaemia and which appear to bind to PTH receptors, but which do not cross-react with PTH in immunoassays. A number of these peptides do, however, show considerable homologies in the amino acid composition of the aminoterminal fragment of PTH responsible for binding to the PTH receptor. These peptides may therefore be responsible for the majority of cases of HHM arising in patients with solid tumours (Ralston 1987).

Treatment of hypercalcaemia involves the management of the underlying tumour and may include surgical excision, irradiation or the use of cytotoxic drugs. Hormonal therapy may also be appropriate, particularly for carcinoma of the breast or prostate. Direct treatment of skeletal metastases occasionally exacerbates the biochemical disturbance (Legha et al. 1981). The life expectancy of the patients is usually short so that specific measures directed at hypercalcaemia are usually only necessary when this is severe. These are dealt with below.

Other Causes of Hypercalcaemia

A list of other causes of hypercalcaemia is shown in Table 7.2. Most of the other causes of hypercalcaemia are relatively uncommon in old age, but two exceptions are those of vitamin D intoxication and treatment with thiazide diuretics. The former is usually due to the unsupervised treatment of osteomalacia with large repeated doses of calciferol, but may also occur during follow-up treatment of iatrogenic hypoparathyroidism after neck surgery (Paterson 1980). Problems can also arise with the inappropriate use of the vitamin D derivative alfacalcidol (1,2 hydroxycholecaciferol) in the management of osteoporosis or osteomalacia. Since alfacalcidol is not dependent upon renal metabolism for its hypercalcaemic effect, close monitoring is required to avoid dangerous rises in the serum calcium concentration. The drug has a place in the management of hypoparathyroidism and renal osteodystrophy. However, its efficacy in osteoporosis has not been established, and it is no more effective than calciferol in the treatment of osteomalacia.

Familial benign hypercalcaemia has no effect on life expectancy (Law and Heath 1985).

Table 7.2. Causes of hypercalcaemia

Primary hyperparathyroidism
Hypercalcaemia of malignancy
Thiazide diuretics
Vitamin D toxicity
Immobility – Paget's disease
Hyperthyroidism
Familial hypocalciuric (benign) hypercalcaemia
Sarcoidosis
Milk–alkali syndrome
Tertiary hyperparathyroidism

Severe Hypercalcaemia

In an elderly patient this is most likely to be caused by malignancy or primary hyperparathyroidism although vitamin D intoxication may on occasion be the cause. The symptoms are those of vomiting and abdominal pain, progressing to depression of consciousness. The patient may also be dehydrated, hypotensive and pyrexial. Electrolyte and fluid loss is the result of vomiting, and failure of renal tubular concentration mechanisms. The serum calcium concentration is often greater than 4 mmol/l.

The mainstay of treatment is vigorous correction of the extracellular fluid volume depletion. Intravenous normal saline is required and up to 5 l may be necessary in the first 24 h with potassium and magnesium supplements being added (Hosking 1983).

Stimulation of calciuresis using frusemide may be considered once the patient has been rehydrated, but large and frequent doses of frusemide are required (120 mg three-hourly) and this can cause a serious electrolyte imbalance.

There has been considerable recent interest in the use of disphosphonates to inhibit bone resorption and calcium mobilisation in hypercalcaemia of malignancy. The newer agents such as aminohydroxypropylidene bisphosphonate appear to have great therapeutic promise in this area but are not yet available for general use. Etidronate disodium has, however, now been licensed for this indication and appears to be of value. The drug must be used intravenously and current dosage recommendations are 7.5 mg/kg by slow intravenous infusion on three successive days after the patient has been adequately rehydrated. Calcitonin may have additive effects with etidronate and the drugs should be used together in severe cases. Maintenance therapy with oral etidronate may be considered in patients in whom specific antitumour therapy is not feasible.

In cases where there is increased calcium resorption from bone, calcitonin should be administered to suppress the resorption and thus reduce the serum calcium concentration. This produces a fall in serum calcium in most cases and can be rapidly effective. The usual amount of salmon calcitonin is 800–1200 units daily in divided doses, given by subcutaneous intramuscular or occasionally by intravenous injection.

Corticosteroids (prednisolone 40 to 50 mg daily or hydrocortisone 100 mg six-hourly) are useful in hypercalcaemia due to myeloma, vitamin D intoxication or sarcoidosis. They should also be tried if other methods of treating hypercalcaemia due to malignancy have been ineffective, but their effects are less predictable in this situation (Boyle and Fogelman 1980).

In the hypercalcaemia of malignancy, plicamycin (mithramycin) 25 µg/kg body weight by intravenous infusion may have a useful prolonged hypocalcaemic action. However, it can cause marrow toxicity.

If rehydration does not significantly lower serum calcium, if this is greater than 4.5 mmol/l or if there is a cardiac dysrhythmia then the use of intravenous phosphate should be considered. This is given as 500 ml 0.1 M neutral phosphate (disodium or dipotassium) for 8–10 h. This may cause hypotension associated with the precipitation of calcium and phosphate in tissue. The serum calcium continues to fall after the infusion is discontinued. A second infusion of phosphate may be considered after a further 24 h.

In patients presenting with severe hypercalcaemia showing no evidence of malignancy or other specific cause for hypercalcaemia, primary hyperparathyroidism is a likely cause. This diagnosis may be supported by radiographic findings in the hands. These patients ultimately require surgery and, occasionally, despite the anaesthetic risks, an emergency exploration of the neck is indicated. Such patients usually harbour a large and relatively easily located adenoma.

Hypocalcaemia and Hypoparathyroidism

In an elderly patient, hypocalcaemia is most frequently associated with hypoalbuminaemia and hence it is essential that a corrected serum calcium value is calculated. If true hypocalcaemia is documented in an elderly patient, then the possible causes include chronic renal failure, vitamin D deficiency and hypoparathyroidism. Hypoparathyroidism presenting in an elderly patient is almost exclusively due to previous neck surgery such as thyroidectomy or laryngectomy. Though hypoparathyroidism often occurs in the immediate post-operative phase, it may be transient. Again, there are some patients in whom the hypocalcaemia develops insidiously. The initial presentations may be that of tetany or seizures, clinical signs which should alert the doctor to the possibility, as should the scar of previous neck surgery. Calcification of the basal ganglia may show up on a plain skull X-ray and is even more apparent on CT scanning. Hypomagnesaemia may be the cause of hypoparathyroidism and hypocalcaemia. This is seen most commonly in patients with prolonged severe diarrhoeal illness. The typical biochemical findings in hypoparathyroidism are hypocalcaemia and elevated plasma phosphate concentration with normal plasma alkaline phosphatase concentrations. In vitamin D deficiency there is hypocalcaemia with secondary hyperparathyroidism, producing a low plasma phosphate concentration and elevated plasma alkaline phosphatase concentrations and normal renal function. Calcidol concentrations are low.

Treatment of hypoparathyroidism depends on the administration of vitamin D or one of its synthetic hydroxylated analogues such as alphacalcidol or calcitriol. The dose of cholecalciferol required to produce normocalcaemia will be of the order of 200 000 units per day and the effect is gradual in onset. The onset of action of alphacalcidol and calcitriol is much more rapid and therefore more easily adjusted and the dosage ranges for alphacalcidol are 0.5–2.0 μg daily and for calcitriol, 1–3 μg daily. In such patients regular monitoring of the serum calcium is essential to prevent overdosage and hypercalcaemia, and long-term follow-up is essential.

References

Adams P, Davies GT, Sweetman P (1970) Osteoporosis and the effects of ageing on bone mass in elderly men and women. Q J Med 39: 602–615

Aldinger KA, Hickey RC, Ibanez M et al. (1982) Parathyroid carcinoma: a clinical study of seven cases of functioning and two cases of non functioning parathyroid cancer. Cancer 49: 388–399

Boyd JC, Ladenson JH (1984) Value of laboratory tests in the differential diagnosis of hypercalcaemia. Am J Med 77: 863–872

Boyle IT, Fogelman I (1980) Glucocorticosteroids and oestrogens in the management of hypercalcaemia. Metab Bone 2: 203–206

Burns J, Paterson CR (1985) Single dose vitamin D treatment for osteomalacia in the elderly. Br Med J 290: 281–282

Burns J, Davidson AV, MacLennan WJ, Paterson CR (1985) The value of serum 25-hydroxyvitamin D assays in screening elderly patients for vitamin D deficiency. J Clin Exp Gerontol 2: 213–222

Chestnut CH, Ivey JL, Gruber HE et al. (1983) Stanazolol in postmenopausal osteoporosis: therapeutic efficacy and possible mechanism of action. Metabolism 32: 571–580

Christiansen C (1982) Prevention and treatment of postmenopausal osteoporosis. In: Menezel J, Robin GC, Makin M, Steinberg R (eds) Osteoporosis. Wiley, Chichester, pp 373–384

Christiansen C, Christiansen M, Richo P et al. (1981) Effect of 1, 25 dihydroxyvitamin D3 itself or combined with hormone treatment in preventing postmenopausal osteoporosis. Eur J Clin Invest 11: 305–309

Cook PJ, Exton-Smith AN, Brocklehurst JC et al. (1982) Fractured femurs, falls and bone disorders. J R Coll Physicians Lond 16: 45–49

Corless D, Dawson E, Fraser F et al. (1985) Do vitamin D supplements improve the physical capabilities of elderly hospital patients? Age Ageing 14: 76–84

Davies M, Mawer EB, Hann JT, Stephens WP, Taylor JL (1985) Vitamin D prophyllaxis in the elderly: a simple method suitable for large populations. Age Ageing 14: 349–354

Devgun MS, Paterson CR, Cohen C et al. (1980) Possible value of fluorescent lighting in the prevention of vitamin D deficiency in the elderly. Age and Ageing 9: 117–120

Exton-Smith AN, Milland PH, Payne PR et al. (1969) Pattern of development of loss of bone with age. Lancet 2: 1154–1157

Feest TG, Wand MK, Ellis HA et al. (1977) Renal bone disease – what is it and why does it happen? Clin Endocrinol (Suppl 7): 195–235

Findling JW, Adams ND, Lemann J et al. (1982) Vitamin D metabolites and parathyroid hormone in Cushing's syndrome: relationship to calcium and phosphorus homeostasis. J Clin Endocrinol Metab 54: 1039–1044

Fraser SA, Anderson JB, Smith DA, Wilson GM (1971) Osteoporosis and fractures following thyrotoxicosis. Lancet 1: 981–983

Hackeng WHL, Lips P, Netelenbos JC, Lips CJM (1986) Clinical implications of estimation of intact parathyroid hormone (PTH) versus total immunoreactive PTH in normal subjects and hyperparathyroid patients. J Clin Endocrinol Metab 63: 447–453

Hahn TJ (1978) Corticosteroid-induced osteopoenia. Arch Intern Med 138: 882–885

Heaney RP, Gallagher JC, Johnson CC et al. (1982) Calcium nutrition and bone health in the elderly. Am J Clin Nutr 30: 1603–1611

Heath D, Melton LJ, Chu CP (1980) Diabetes mellitus and risk of skeletal fracture. New Eng J Med 303: 567–570

Heath DA, Wright AD, Barnes AD et al. (1980) Surgical treatment of primary hyperparathyroidism in the elderly. Br Med J 280: 1406–1408

Hodkinson HM, Hodkinson I (1980) Range for 25-hydroxyvitamin D in elderly subjects in whom osteomalacia has been excluded on histological and biochemical criteria. J Clin Exp Gerontol 2: 133–140

Hodkinson I, Hodkinson HM (1981) Normal range for osteoid in iliac crest bone of elderly subjects assessed by bright line counting. J Clin Exp Gerontol 3: 127–134

Hosking DJ (1980) Treatment of severe hypercalcaemia with calcitriol. Metab Bone 2: 207–212

Hosking DJ (1983) Disequilibrium hypercalcaemia. Br Med J 286: 326–327

Jowsey J, Deterbeck LC (1969) The importance of thyroid hormones to bone metabolism and calcium homeostasis. Endocrinology 85: 87–95

Jowsey J, Riggs BL (1970) Bone formation in hypercortisonism. Acta Endocrinol (Copenh) 63: 21–28

Kanis JA, Grilland-Cumming DF, Russell REE (1982) Comparative physiology and pharmacology of the metabolites and analogues of vitamin D. In: Parsons JA (ed) Endocrinology of calcium metabolism. Raven Press, New York, pp 321–362

Knowelden J, Buhr AJ, Dunbar O (1964) Incidence of fractures in persons over 35 years of age. Br J Prev Soc Med 18: 130–141

Krubsack AJ, Wilson SD, Lawson TL et al. (1986) Prospective comparison of radionuclide computed tomographic and sonographic localisation of parathyroid tumours. World J Surg 10: 579–585

Law WM, Heath H (1985) Familial benign hypercalcaemia. Ann Intern Med 102: 511–519

Legha SS, Powell K, Buzdar AU et al. (1981) Tamoxifen-induced hypercalcaemia in breast cancer. Cancer 47: 2803–2806

Levin ME, Boiseau VC, Avioli LV (1976) Effects of diabetes mellitus on bone mass in juvenile and adult-onset diabetes. New Engl J Med 294: 241–244

MacLennan WJ (1979) Vitamin D metabolism in the elderly. J Clin Exp Gerontol 1: 1–11

MacLennan WJ, Hamilton JC (1977) Vitamin D supplements and 25-hydroxyvitamin D concentrations in the elderly. Br Med J 2: 859–861

MacLennan WJ, Hamilton JC, Timothy JJ (1979) 25-hydroxyvitamin D concentration in old people living at home. J Clin Nutr 36: 1014–1031

Matkovic V, Kostial K, Simenovik I et al. (1979) Bone status and fracture rate in two regions of Yugoslavia. Am J Clin Nutr 27: 916–925

Mazzoli GF, Passeri M, Gennari C et al. (1986) Effects of salmon calcitonin in post menopausal osteoporosis: a controlled double-blind clinical study. Calcif Tissue Int 38: 3–8

Mundy GR, Martin TJ (1982) The hypercalcaemia of malignancy: pathogenesis and management. Metabolism 31: 1247–1277

Nordin BEC, Peacock M, Aaron J et al. (1980) Osteoporosis and osteomalacia. Clin Endocrol Metab 9: 177–205

Nordin BEC, Baker MLR, Horsman A, Peacock M (1985) A prospective trial of the effects of vitamin D supplementation on metacarpal bone loss in elderly women. Am J Clin Nutr 42: 470–474

Omdahl JL, Garry PJ, Hunsaker LA et al. (1982) Nutritional status in a healthy elderly population: vitamin D. Am J Clin Nutr 36: 1225–1233

Palmer M, Adami HO, Bergstrom R, Jakobsson S, Akerstrom G, Lyinghall S (1987) Survival and renal function in untreated hypercalcaemia. Lancet 1: 59–62

Parfitt AM, Gallagher JC, Heaney et al. (1982) Vitamin D and bone health in the elderly. Am J Clin Nutr 36: 1014–1031

Paterson CR (1980) Vitamin D poisoning: survey of causes in 21 patients with hypercalcaemia. Lancet 1: 1164–1166

Paterson CR, MacLennan WJ (1984) Bone disease in the elderly. Wiley, Chichester

Paterson CR, Burns J, Mowat E (1984) Long term follow up of untreated primary hyperparathyroidism. Br Med J 289: 1261–1263

Ralston SH (1987) The pathogenesis of humoural hypercalcaemia of malignancy. Lancet 2: 1443–1446

Rhis B, Thomson K, Christiansen C (1987) Does calcium supplementation prevent postmenopausal bone loss? New Engl J Med 316: 173–177

Riggs BL, Seeman E, Hodgson SJ et al. (1982) Effect of the fluoride/calcium regimen on vertebral fracture occurrence in postmenopausal osteoporosis. New Engl J Med 306: 446–450

Schott GD, Wills MR (1976) Muscle weakness in osteomalacia. Lancet 1: 626–629

Stanbury SW (1981) Vitamin D and hyperparathyroidism. J R Coll Physicians Lond 15: 205–217

Stevenson JC, Whitehead MI (1982) Postmenopausal osteoporosis. Br Med J 285: 585–587

Taggart HM, Appelbaum-Bouden D, Haffen S et al. (1982) Reduction in high density lipoprotein by anabolic steroid (Stanazolol) therapy for postmenopausal osteoporosis. Metabolism 31: 1147–1152

Tibblin S, Palsson N, Rydberg J (1983) Hyperparathyroidism in the elderly. Ann Surg 197: 135–138

Wigzell FW, Alan AKMS, MacLennan WJ et al. (1981) Osteomalacia and kyphosis. J Clin Exp Gerontol 3: 161–194

8 Pituitary and Adrenal Disorders

Pituitary Tumours and Hypopituitarism

Disorders of the anterior pituitary gland, until recently, were considered to be rare in the elderly. This was due in part to a lack of interest in the clinical problems of the elderly, and to the fact that the features of pituitary dysfunction may be difficult to distinguish from those of ageing. More careful scrutiny has revealed that they do occur, but that the effects of ageing and multiple pathology often modify their presentation.

Pituitary Tumours

Autopsy studies of old people have found that pituitary adenomas are common, occurring in 13% of patients over the age of 80 (Kovacs et al. 1980). Most of these are microadenomas occupying between 5% and 10% of the total anterior pituitary mass. Around half contain significant concentrations of prolactin, whereas a few produce ACTH, FSH, LH or TSH, and the remainder are undifferentiated chromophobe tumours.

These microadenomas have minimal effects. Around one in five are associated with radiological evidence of an enlarged sella turcica, but this is comparable with sellar enlargement in 18% of patients with "normal" pituitaries (Burrow et al. 1981). Headaches and visual symptoms are rare.

There is little epidemiological information on the prevalence of clinically obvious pituitary adenoma in old age, but the general belief is that this is low. Certainly, an analysis of cases of chromophobe adenomas presenting at regional neurological centres demonstrated that most cases occurred around the age of 40; and that the numbers over the age of 60 were less than one-sixth of this (Banna 1976). Since the numbers showed a sharp decline after the age of 40, it is unlikely that this distribution simply represents a reluctance to treat and investigate elderly patients.

Older patients with pituitary tumours tend to present late with tumours which cause local pressure effects, particularly visual failure and often hypopituitarism. Recent evidence demonstrated that a substantial proportion of apparently non-functioning pituitary macroadenomas, particularly in men, are capable of synthesising and sometimes secreting FSH, and less frequently LH or subunits. Ten of 37 such patients were aged over 65 years (Kilbanski 1987). The majority did not secrete intact LH and therefore had normal or subnormal testosterone levels often associated with secondary hypogonadism. Occasionally, LH-beta-subunits cross-react with the LH assay to suggest an increase in the serum LH concentrations (Snyder 1987).

Acromegaly is occasionally seen in elderly patients, who usually have had long-standing growth hormone hypersecretion manifesting itself in the facial appearance. Patients also suffer the long-term cardiovascular effects of growth hormone hypersecretion such as hypertension, cardiac enlargement, ischaemic heart disease and heart failure.

Chromophobe adenomas secreting prolactin are likely to present with local pressure effects but the symptoms and signs of hypogonadism may be accentuated in an elderly male. Hypersecretion of ACTH from a pituitary chromophobe adenoma causing Nelson's syndrome (without previous adrenalectomy) has been reported in old age (Sterling and Hall 1979).

Thyrotrophin (TSH) secreting pituitary tumours are extremely rare, but can occur in elderly patients. They may present with both a goitre and hyperthyroidism and there may be clinical evidence of hypersecretion of other anterior pituitary hormones, particularly growth hormone. Such patients have measurable or elevated serum TSH concentrations, in contrast to the patients with primary hyperthyroidism in whom TSH is suppressed. They also secrete excessive amounts of TSH alpha-subunit. The pituitary fossa is usually enlarged (Smallridge 1987).

The assessment of anterior pituitary hormone secretion is summarised in Chap. 12. In a patient with hyperprolactinaemia it is important to rule out other causes such as drug side-effects (phenothiazines, haloperidol, metoclopramide or reserpine), chronic renal failure, and hypothyroidism. It is important to identify not only hormone hypersecretion but also evidence of deficiencies of other anterior pituitary hormones, particularly ACTH and TSH. Large tumours may cause posterior pituitary failure with diabetes insipidus.

The pituitary fossa is likely to be enlarged on X-rays in patients with macroadenomas. High resolution CT scanning has added much to the investigation of hypothalamic pituitary disease, both in the identification of macroadenomas and in assessing supra- and infrasellar extension of larger tumours. Accurate plotting of the visual fields is also important in the initial evaluation and follow-up of pituitary tumours.

The management of patients with pituitary adenomas depends on whether the tumours are functional, causing hormone hypersecretion, or non-functional, causing local pressure effects. An initial approach may be to give bromocriptine. Even large prolactin-secreting macroadenomas often respond to bromocriptine with a decline in prolactin secretion and reduction in tumour size, and this is often sufficient to reverse significant visual field defects. Once this occurs, a small maintained dose of bromocriptine in the order of 2.5–7.5 mg per day is often sufficient to prevent relapse. An alternative, once bromocriptine has achieved tumour shrinkage, is to apply external pituitary radiation. Though the effects of radiation are gradual they are usually sufficient to prevent tumour regrowth and allow gradual withdrawal of bromocriptine therapy. Irradiation may lead to hypopituitarism, but this is less of a problem in an elderly patient with a limited lifespan than in a younger individual.

Growth hormone hypersecretion in patients with acromegaly may also respond to bromocriptine, but the response is usually incomplete and, to even achieve this, much larger doses of the order of 20 mg bromocriptine daily are required. It is important to increase the dose of bromocriptine very gradually as side-effects such as confusion, dizziness, postural hypotension, and nausea are frequent.

Since patients with acromegaly often show an inadequate response to bromo-criptine, they are frequently exposed to alternative remedies. One of these is external irradiation but this only produces a gradual reduction in hormone levels. However, the main problem associated with growth hormone hypersecretion in old age is cardiac enlargement and dysfunction, and this is unlikely to improve even if there is a dramatic decline in hormone secretion. Irradiation may then pro-vide an adequate response rate. Long-acting somatostatin analogues administered by injection are currently under evaluation in acromegaly and appear to be effec-tive at inhibiting GH hypersecretion. These can be self-administered by patients, the frequency being twice or three daily for Sandostatin.

Surgery should be reserved for elderly patients who are intolerant of other therapies or suffer from local pressure effects, particularly those on the visual pathways. Unless the tumour is particularly extensive, trans-sphenoidal surgery is usually practicable even if there is some suprasellar extension of the tumour. Patients with non-functional tumours usually present with local pressure effects, and are likely to require surgical intervention. If the tumour is particularly exten-sive, trans-sphenoidal surgery may not be possible and transfrontal surgery may be necessary. This should be followed by external pituitary radiation to prevent tumour recurrence.

Anterior Pituitary Hormone Deficiency

There is no information on the prevalence of hypopituitarism in old age, but case reports in the medical literature and clinical experience of endocrinologists suggest that this is not infrequent if looked for carefully (Belchetz 1985). Though there are many potential causes of hypopituitarism in elderly patients, many, after extensive investigation, have no apparent cause. It has been suggested that such patients have auto-immune hypophysitis, but it is more likely that the condition is related to local vascular disease. In a proportion of cases, there may be a history of post-partum haemorrhage in a pregnancy with a failure of lactation (Sheehan's syndrome). The condition may also follow acute vascular insufficiency, and infarc-tion of a pituitary tumour may also be involved (Markowitz et al. 1981). This causes pituitary apoplexy, which often simulates subarachnoid haemorrhage, with the dramatic features of headache, vomiting, truchal rigidity, drowsiness, visual loss, hemiparesis and focal neurological signs including cranial nerve palsies. Sometimes the clinical picture is less clearly defined (Sachdev et al. 1981). In this situation and particularly in an elderly patient with multiple pathology, the condition may be missed, and only identified later when the patient presents with chronic pituitary insufficiency.

In old age, hypopituitarism often has an insidious onset (Belchetz 1985). Common clinical features in old age include pallor, a thin skin with a fine texture, absence of body hair, signs of hypothyroidism, and postural hypotension. All of these signs are of course common in old people with normal pituitary thyroid and adrenal function, so laboratory investigations are frequently negative.

The most useful initial screening tests are the serum sodium and serum thyroid hormone concentrations. Both are usually low. Confirmatory investigations include a low basal serum TSH concentration with a reduced TSH response to TRH. It is particularly important to measure the basal cortisol level and its response to Synacthen. Further stimulatory testing may be necessary (Chap. 12). X-rays of the pituitary fossa may point towards an underlying pituitary tumour.

Initial treatment involves replacement therapy with thyroxine and glucocorticoids and, if both deficiencies are present, it is important that glucocorticoid therapy is instituted before thyroxine is given. The latter given alone may precipitate a hyperadrenal crisis. Glucocorticoid replacement may sometimes unmask posterior pituitary failure with vasopressin deficiency and cause the sudden onset of diabetes insipidus. This is particularly likely to occur in patients with large pituitary tumours or lesions of the hypothalamus.

Disorders of the Adrenal Glands

Glucocorticoid Secretion

Illness and Adreno-cortical Function

A variety of physical and mental disorders which are common in old age have an important effect on adrenal function. An example is that old people with a fractured proximal femur have a more prolonged elevation of plasma cortisol levels than young patients with severe injury (Frayn et al. 1983). The precise explanation for the elevation is unclear, but if a similar change occurs in other forms of infection or injury in old age it could have an important negative effect on the rate of resolution of infection or wound healing. An important caveat is that another study found that relatively healthy old people undergoing a herniorrhaphy showed post-operative plasma cortisol levels which were similar to those of young adults (Amety 1985). It may be that poor health, rather than chronological age, is the main determinant of changes in adrenal function.

Depression also has an effect on pituitary-adrenal function, causing hypersecretion of cortisol and interfering with feedback inhibition of the pituitary. Evidence for this is that a 1 mg oral dose of dexamethasone given at 11.00 p.m. has no depressive effect on the plasma cortisol level measured at 4.00 p.m. the following day. In a general psychiatric population, the test was abnormal in 43% of patients with depression, and 96% of patients with an abnormal test had depression (Carroll et al. 1981). Unfortunately, the test is also abnormal in around half of elderly patients with dementia (Spar and Gorner 1982). This means that it provides clinicians with little help in the difficult task of distinguishing a reversible depressive disorder from irreversible senile or multi-infarct dementia.

Cushing's Disease and Syndrome – Hypercortisolism

Excessive secretion of glucocorticoids is most often due to bilateral adrenal hyperplasia, occasionally to a secreting adrenal adenoma, and rarely to adrenal carcinoma. Bilateral adrenal hyperplasia is usually secondary to excessive ACTH secretion from the pituitary gland (Cushing's disease) but up to 15% of cases are secondary to ectopic ACTH secretion. In the elderly, the latter most commonly emanates from a small cell carcinoma of bronchus, whereas in younger patients it is more likely to be the result of a slow-growing bronchial carcinoid or pancreatic tumour. A variant of bilateral adrenal hyperplasia characterised by the development of adrenal cortical nodules (which may be autonomous) – nodular hyperplasia – is also recognised. Finally, as in younger patients, Cushing's syndrome in the elderly may be iatrogenic, due to excessive glucocorticoid treatment for another pathology such as rheumatoid arthritis.

There have been no major studies of Cushing's syndrome in the elderly, but, in one very large series, 5% of patients were over the age of 60 (Nakai 1984). A review of patients with an age range of 7–58 suggested that ageing may have a variety of effects (Urbanic and George 1981). Older patients are less likely to develop the typical livid cutaneous striae, possibly because of changes in the chemical and physical properties of ageing connective tissue. Again, truncal obesity is of less diagnostic value in old age, where changes in energy balance produce an increased percentage body fat. Other features are more common in older patients. Thus an age-related decline in muscle power means that old people are more likely to present with a proximal myopathy. There also is an increased prevalence of cardiac disease and hypertension. A reduced renal reserve means they are more likely to develop fluid retention. Osteoporosis and back pain are frequent findings in Cushing's syndrome and this is likely to be particularly important in the osteoporotic skeletons of older patients. In one survey, osteoporosis was more commonly associated with severe bone rarefaction in men than women (Urbanic and George 1981). Depression, while frequent in hypercortisolism, is also common in the elderly.

The presentation of Cushing's syndrome, due to ectopic ACTH production by a non-pituitary tumour such as bronchial carcinoma, differs from typical Cushing's syndrome. More common presenting features are cachexia, progressive muscle weakness, hypertension, carbohydrate intolerance and hypokalaemia. The disease usually follows a rapid down-hill course.

When a diagnosis of Cushing's syndrome is considered, it is important to remember that alcohol abuse may cause a pseudo Cushing's syndrome with a plethoric face, obesity and hypercortisolism. This usually resolves quickly on abstention. Obese patients with depression may also cause diagnostic difficulties, and have rather more persistent abnormalities of cortisol secretion.

The investigation of patients with suspected Cushing's syndrome and hypercortisolism is detailed in Chap. 12. Elderly patients are frequently taking drug therapy for other disorders and some of these may interfere with investigations. Spironolactone interferes with the fluorometric assay of cortisol, while enzyme-inducing drugs such as anticonvulsants and rifampicin may induce the hepatic metabolism of dexamethasone and thus obscure the effects of suppression testing.

In the past, patients with pituitary-dependent Cushing's disease were treated by bilateral adrenalectomy, but this left them with the long-term risk of developing Nelson's syndrome, a condition caused by excessive ACTH secretion from a pituitary tumour. Treatment is now directed at the pituitary gland itself, in which 50%–85% of patients have a basophilic pituitary microadenoma, but up to 25% have no discrete tumour and a few will have a macroadenoma. In a few centres with the necessary expertise, trans-sphenoidal selective adenomectomy gives impressive results with a high proportion of remissions from hypercortisolism and a low post-operative incidence of pituitary hormone deficiency. The 5-year recurrence rate of Cushing's disease is only 5%. The results of resecting macroadenomas are less impressive and the prognosis for large tumours is poor.

The condition can also be treated by using yttrium or gold rods implanted via the transnasal route under general anaesthesia to irradiate the pituitary. Though the procedure gives good results, it is practised in only a few centres. Megavoltage external irradiation to the pituitary eliminates hypercortisolism in up to 50% of patients, but the treatment takes several years to work. Since rapid control of hypercortisolism is desirable, irradiation should be combined with medical therapy. An alternative is to combine irradiation with bilateral adrenalectomy to prevent the subsequent development of Nelson's syndrome.

Medical therapy may be directed to blocking corticosteroid synthesis (Howlett et al. 1985). Metyrapone achieves this by inhibiting the enzyme 11-betahydroxylase. This can be used as primary treatment, or to induce clinical remission of the hypercortisolism, prior to definitive pituitary or adrenal surgery, or while awaiting the effects of pituitary radiotherapy. It is also useful in correcting endocrine abnormality in patients who are psychiatrically or physically ill secondary to the hypercortisolism. The adrenolytic drug ap'-DDD (mitotane) is also effective but has significant toxicity, while aminoglutethimide, another enzyme blocking drug, is poorly tolerated. There is currently significant interest in the use of ketoconazole, an antifungal drug which blocks corticosteroid synthesis.

Bromocriptine has been used to reduce ACTH hypersecretion and hypercortisolism in a subgroup of patients whose pituitary adenoma is of neurointermediate lobe origin (Lamberts et al. 1982). Both cyproheptadine and sodium valproate have induced remission in a proportion of patients with Cushing's disease or Nelson's syndrome, but experience with these agents remains limited.

If a patient has an adrenal adenoma or carcinoma, then definitive surgery should be performed, ideally after normalising the metabolic state and hypercorticolism with metyrapone. Elderly patients with ectopic ACTH secretion due to a non-pituitary tumour such as a bronchial carcinoma have a very poor prognosis. It may be possible to stabilise the metabolic state using metyrapone or one of the other drugs active on the adrenal cortex. This allows time for more definitive therapy at the primary tumour. Many of these patients, however, are resistant to the effects of metyropone and other agents and their life expectancy is generally of the order of weeks.

Primary Adrenocortical Insufficiency (Addison's Disease)

Addison's disease implies failure of both glucocorticoid (cortisol) and mineralocorticoid (aldosterone) production. It has a peak prevalence in early middle age but is also encountered in the elderly (Mason et al. 1968) (Table 8.1). In old age, similar proportions of cases are due to auto-immune adrenalitis and tuberculosis (Moss et al. 1983). Adrenal failure due to carcinomatosis is less frequent and other pathologies such as sarcoidosis and amyloidosis are extremely rare.

Table 8.1. Prevalence per 1 000 000 of Addison's disease (Mason et al. 1968)

Age (years)	Tuberculous disease	Non-tuberculous disease
0–24	0.9	4.7
25–44	13.8	34.4
45–64	15.4	22.6
65–69	0	13.5
>70	4.0	4.0

Many of the clinical features of the disorder such as weakness, lethargy, weight loss, anorexia, hypotension, vomiting or diarrhoea are either vague or non-specific. These are common in frail elderly patients where they are rarely due to adrenal disease. A more useful sign is that of hyperpigmentation, particularly where the buccal membranes or flexor creases are involved. Patients may have a non-specific anaemia. Plasma abnormalities, usually, but not always, associated with the disorder include a low or low normal plasma sodium with a high normal or high plasma potassium. There is usually a degree of uraemia with a mild metabolic acidosis and, occasionally, hypercalcaemia. Definitive investigations for establishing the diagnosis and differentiating primary from the secondary adreno-cortical failure are summarised in Chap. 12. An X-ray of the abdomen may show evidence of adrenal calcification.

Most patients with tuberculous adrenal insufficiency have radiological evidence of tuberculosis. In old people with tuberculosis the 1/10 000 dilution of tuberculin often gives a negative skin reaction, but at a dilution of 1/1000 this is usually positive. There is often no history of tuberculosis, and, if there is, this may have occurred 10–20 years previously, so the infection is no longer active.

Around 75% of patients with non-tuberculous Addison's disease have adrenal antibodies in their sera (Nerup 1974). Even in old age these occur in less than 0.2% of control subjects. Around half of patients also have thyroid antibodies in their sera, while one-fifth have gastric parietal cell antibodies.

A significant proportion of women with Addison's disease may also have or develop primary hypothyroidism. It has also been reported that patients with newly diagnosed Addison's disease may have an elevated serum TSH which reverts to normal with cortisol replacement. These patients may, or may not, have a low serum thyroxine and lack antithyroid antibodies. A diagnosis of primary hypothyroidism should not therefore be made until adequate hydrocortisone therapy has been instituted and the patient's condition stabilised. In addition, thyroxine therapy should never be instituted prior to hydrocortisone, as this increases the metabolic rate of cortisol and can precipitate a hypoadrenal crisis.

Elderly patients are usually adequately controlled by 20–30 mg daily of hydrocortisone in two divided doses, say 20 mg in the morning, and 10 mg around the time of the evening meal. If, despite this, hypotension, postural hypotension, hyponatraemia or hyperkalaemia persists, then fluorocortisone should be added in an initial dose of 50 μg daily, its efficacy being monitored by its effect on the blood pressure and electrolytes. During infections and other acute illnesses or intercurrent stress, the dose of hydrocortisone should be doubled. If the patient is vomiting, hydrocortisone should be administered parenterally. Treatment with enzyme-inducing drugs such as rifampicin, which increase the metabolic clearance rate of hydrocortisone, may also increase hydrocortisone requirements.

Should a patient with Addison's disease develop an Addisonian crisis during an intercurrent illness or stress, this should be managed with saline to replace electrolytes, and intravenous hydrocortisone. Dextrose is also given if the patient is hypoglycaemic (Burke 1980).

Primary Hyperaldosteronism

In this condition there is excessive secretion of aldosterone by the zona glomerulosa of the adrenal cortex. It is rare, occurring in less than 1% of hypertensive patients (Ferris et al. 1981). The mean age of diagnosis in patients with the disorder identified at a hypertension clinic was 48, with 95% confidence limits between 26 and 70 (Grim 1979). However, the low upper age limit may reflect a reluctance to investigate for the condition in extreme old age. About two-thirds of cases are due to an aldosterone-producing adrenocortical adenoma; one-third to bilateral glomerulosa hyperplasia, and a few to an adrenocortical carcinoma.

The main clinical feature of the disorder is hypertension, usually associated with a low serum potassium concentration. However, in hypertensive elderly patients, hypokalaemia is far more likely to be due to either diuretic therapy or secondary hyperaldosteronism. There also is a small proportion of patients (10%) with primary hyperaldosteronism who have a normal serum potassium concentration. As a consequence, the serum potassium concentration produces too many false positive and negative results for it to be a useful screening test (Streeten et al. 1979). A reasonable approach would be only to investigate hypertensive patients for hyperaldosteronism if they have hypokalaemia not related to an obvious cause such as diuretic therapy, or patients with normokalaemia whose hypertension responds inadequately to conventional antihypertensive agents.

Primary hyperaldosteronism is associated with a low plasma renin activity. Low renin hypertension, however, is frequent in the elderly and rarely associated with primary hyperaldosteronism (Messerli et al. 1983).

The investigation of patients suspected of having primary hyperaldosteronism is detailed in Chap. 12.

The treatment of adrenocorticol adenoma causing hyperaldosteronism is clearcut with unilateral adrenalectomy normalising blood pressure in 70% of patients and restoring potassium balance in all (Melby 1985). If the condition is long-standing then there may be irreversible changes in the kidneys which perpetuate the hypertension. The likely efficacy of surgery in normalising blood pressure can be predicted by the blood pressure response to spironolactone in a dose 300–400 µg daily for 4–6 weeks. Whether surgery will produce such satisfactory results in elderly patients is unclear. If the primary hyperaldosteronism is due to idiopathic bilateral glomerular hyperplasia, then the treatment of choice is spironolactone and unilateral adrenalectomy is contra-indicated.

It may, therefore, be reasonable in elderly patients with primary hyperaldosteronism, to treat them all with spironolactone, as the risks that a patient is harbouring an adrenocortical carcinoma are very low and in any case other features may point to this diagnosis. Amiloride is an effective alternative to spironolactone. If additional antihypertensive therapy is necessary, especially for patients with idiopathic bilateral glomerular hyperplasia, then angiotensin converting enzyme inhibitors appear to be particularly effective (Melby 1985). Nifedipine may also be useful (Nadler et al. 1985).

In summary, the incidence of primary hyperaldosteronism as a cause of hypertension in the elderly is unknown. When the condition is diagnosed, the patient can probably be satisfactorily managed with spironolactone and other antihypertensive agents. It is difficult, therefore, to justify performing expensive and time-consuming tests to diagnose this condition.

Diseases of the Adrenal Medulla

Although there is an age-related increase in plasma noradrenaline and total catecholamine levels, these are no higher in hypertensive than in normotensive old people (Lake et al. 1977). This suggests that increased sympathetic activity is not a major cause of hypertension in old age. Since plasma renin and aldosterone levels are reduced in elderly hypertensive patients, it seems likely that hypertension in this group is usually the result of reduced vascular impedance associated with atherosclerosis or changes in the structure of connective tissue (Messerli et al. 1983).

Phaeochromocytoma

Though the condition occurs in only 1.35/100 000 individuals per year, around half the cases occur in patients over the age of 60 (Beard et al. 1983) (Table 8.2). This means that in a catchment area with a total population of 200 000 at least one case of phaeochromocytoma is likely to be encountered in an elderly patient each year.

The condition may simply present as sustained hypertension but paroxysmal symptoms are common (Goldfien 1981). These are characterised by headache, sweating, palpitations, anxiety, tremor, nausea, visual disturbances and chest or

Table 8.2. Phaeochromocytoma-autopsy series (Sutton et al. 1981)

Age (years)	Number of patients
0–19	4
20–39	7
40–59	19
60–79	20
80+	4

abdominal discomfort. Their frequency varies between once every few months to many times a day. A clear and carefully taken history is required to distinguish these episodes from symptoms due to an anxiety neurosis, thyrotoxicosis or depression. This may present problems in an elderly patient who has an intellectual deficit or a communication problem.

Apart from hypertension, the clinical symptoms and signs may be non-specific and may include cachexia and excessive sweating. Patients are often mildly hyperglycaemic. Rarely, a mass is palpable in the abdomen. Investigation of the condition is detailed in Chap. 12.

Even if surgery is contemplated, the condition should initially be stabilised by medical means for at least 14 days pre-operatively. The mainstay of treatment is the alpha-adrenergic antagonist phenoxybenzamine, given in an initial dose of 10 mg twice daily, increasing this by 10 mg every 2–3 days until hypertension is controlled without severe postural hypotension. This drug has a long half-life and accumulation may be a problem in an elderly patient. Propranolol may be necessary to induce beta-adrenoceptor blockade and control a tachycardia or tachydysrhythmia. If invasive investigations such as angiography are considered, then full alpha- and, if necessary, beta-adrenoceptor blockade should be instituted prior to these. The vasoconstrictor effects of catecholamines often cause a serious volume depletion and when phenoxybenzamine is instituted there is a rapid expansion in blood volume with a drop in the haematocrit.

The peri-operative care of these patients is most important, and the physician and anaesthetist must exercise a high degree of skill to prevent disastrous fluctuations in blood pressure during the operation. Elderly patients with severe ischaemic heart disease or cerebrovascular disease are unlikely to tolerate surgery and may have to be given less satisfactory long-term medical treatment with phenoxybenzamine or prazosin and propranolol. There may be post-operative problems with hypotension due to down-regulation of adrenoceptors, following prolonged exposure to high circulating catecholamine concentrations.

References

Amety BB (1985) Endocrine reactions during standardised surgical stress: the effects of age and methods of anaesthesia. Age Ageing 14: 96–101

Banna M (1976) Pathology and clinical manifestations. In: Hankinson J, Banna M (eds) Pituitary and parapituitary tumours. Saunders, Philadelphia, pp 13–58

Beard CM, Sheps SG, Kurland LT, Lie JT (1983) Occurrence of phaeochromocytoma in Rochester, Minnesota, 1950 through 1979. Mayo Clin Proc 58: 802–804

Belchetz P (1985) Idiopathic hypopituitarism in the elderly. Br Med J 291: 247–248

Burke CW (1985) Adrenocortical insufficiency. Clin Endocrinol Metab 14: 947–976

Burrow GN, Wortzman G, Rewcastle NG et al. (1981) Microadenomas of the pituitary and sellar tomograms in an unselected autopsy series. N Engl J Med 304: 156–158

Carroll BJ, Feinberg M, Greden JF et al. (1981) A specific laboratory test for the diagnosis of melancholia. Arch Gen Psychiatry 38: 15–22

Ferris JB, Brown JJ, Fraser R et al. (1981) Primary hyperaldosteronism. Clin Endocrinol Metab 10: 419–452

Frayn KN, Stoner HB, Barton RN et al. (1983) Persistence of high plasma glucose, insulin and cortisol concentrations in elderly patients with proximal femoral fractures. Age Ageing 12: 70–76

Grim CE, Weinberger MH, Higgins JT, Kramer NJ (1979) Diagnosis of secondary forms of hypertension. JAMA 237:1331–1335

Goldfien A (1981) Phaeochromocytoma. Clin End Metab 10: 607–630

Howlett TA, Rees LH, Besser GM (1985) Cushing's syndrome. Clin Endocrinol Metab 14: 911-945

Kilbanski A (1987) Non-secreting pituitary tumours. Endocrinol Metab Clin N Am 16: 793–804

Kovacs K, Ryan N, Horvath E et al. (1980) Pituitary adenomas in old age. J Gerontol 35: 16–22

Lake CR, Ziegler MG, Coleman MD, Kopin IJ (1977) Age-adjusted plasma noreprinephine levels are similar in normotensive and hypertensive subjects. N Engl J Med 296: 208–209

Lamberts SWJ, deLange SA, Stefanko SZ (1982) Adrenocorticotrophin-secreting pituitary adenomas originate from the anterior or the intermediate lobe in Cushing's disease: differences in the regulation of hormone secretion. J Clin Endocrinol Metab 54: 286–291

Markowitz S, Sheman L, Kolodry HD, Baruh S (1981) Acute pituitary vascular accident (pituitary apoplexy). Med Clin N Am 65: 105–116

Mason AS, Meade TW, Lee JAH, Morris JV (1968) Epidemiological and clinical picture of Addison's disease. Lancet 2, 744–747

Melby JC (1985) Diagnosis and treatment of primary aldosteronism and isolated hypoaldosteronism. Clin Endocrinol Metab 14: 977–996

Messerli FH, Ventura HO, Glade LB et al. (1983) Essential hypertension in the elderly: haemodynamics, intravascular volume, plasma renin activity and circulating catecholamine levels. Lancet 2: 983–986

Moss CN, England ML, Korval J (1983) Adrenal insufficiency (Addison's disease) in the elderly. J Am Geriatr Soc 33: 63–68

Nadler JL, Hsueh W, Harton R (1985) Therapeutic effect of calcium channel blockade in primary hyperaldosteronism. J Clin Endocrinol Metab 60: 896–899

Nakai (1984) Cushing's disease. In: Belchetz PE (ed) Management of pituitary disease. Chapman and Hall, London, pp 141–157

Nerup J (1974) Addison's disease – serological studies. Acta Endocrinol (Copenh) 76: 142–158

Sachdev Y, Garg VK, Gopal K, Mongia SS (1981) Pituitary apoplexy (spontaneous pituitary necrosis). Postgrad Med J 57: 289–293

Smallridge RC (1987) Thyrotrophin-secreting pituitary tumours. Endocrinol Metab Clin N Am 16: 765–792

Snyder PJ (1987) Gonadotrophin cell pituitary adenomas. Endocrinol Metab Clin N Am 16: 755–764

Spar JE, Gorner R (1982) Does the dexamethasone suppression test distinguish dementia from depression? Am J Psychiatry 139: 238–240

Sterling N, Hall MRP (1979) Chromophobe adenoma of the pituitary with Cushing's syndrome and skin pigmentation. Postgrad Med J 55: 564–566

Streeten DHP, Tomyoz N, Anderson GH (1979) Reliability of screening methods for the diagnosis of primary aldosteronism. Am J Med 67: 403–413

Sutton MG, Sheps SG, Lie JT (1981) Prevalence of clinically unsuspected phaeochromocytoma – review of a 50 year autopsy series. Mayo Clin Proc 56: 354–360

Urbanic RC, George JM (1981) Cushing's disease – 18 years experience. Medicine 60: 14–24

9 Fluid and Electrolyte Imbalance

Fluid and electrolyte homeostasis is dependent upon the integrity of both the endocrine regulatory system and its target organs. The effects of ageing on these are rarely sufficient to cause an imbalance under baseline conditions. However, the gross reduction in their reserve capacities means that relatively minor physiological stresses are often sufficient to cause severe metabolic derangement. There is the further problem that when this does occur, the clinical signs may be vague and non-specific, and go undetected.

Dehydration

The effects of ageing on thirst drive, on posterior pituitary and on renal function mean that old people are at increased risk from dehydration (Chap. 2). These problems may be exacerbated by immobility and mental impairment. Thus a wide range of illnesses including gastro-enteritis, bronchopneumonia and myocardial infarction may all result in a pre-renal uraemia (Leaf 1984). Over-enthusiastic use of diuretics may also cause major problems.

Assessment

The clinical evaluation of fluid imbalance in old age is extremely difficult. A reduction in skin elasticity is indistinguishable from a change in turgor; loss of peri-orbital fat gives the impression of orbital softness; and poor oral hygiene, anti-cholinergic agents, or mouth breathing in chest infections may produce a dry inflamed tongue. Conversely, a patient may be dehydrated (effectively reduced intravascular volume) even if he has a massive ankle oedema. A poor peripheral circulation, a low serum albumin, and increased vascular permeability mean that It may take a long time for a reduced intravascular volume to be corrected from an increased extra vascular compartment. Postural hypotension and failure to fill the neck veins in the supine position remain useful clinical pointers to the presence of dehydration. Drowsiness, confusion or local hypothalamic damage may mask further an already impaired thirst sensation.

If, by virtue of an acute illness, confusion or coma, a patient is at risk of becoming dehydrated, fluid balance should be carefully charted. Nurses, however, may have difficulty in measuring fluid intake in a busy geriatric or general medical ward. They have even greater difficulty in measuring urinary output, particularly if the patient is incontinent and catheterisation is inappropriate. Awareness of the potential for dehydration is therefore essential.

The biochemical changes are more characteristic, consisting of an increased plasma osmolality, an elevated blood urea and, usually, an increased serum sodium concentration. The effects of ageing on renal function result in the urinary osmolality being normal or only slightly elevated. Pre-existing anaemia and hypoproteinaemia may lessen the validity of haematocrit and serum protein concentrations as indices of dehydration.

Treatment

Caution should be observed in replacing fluid. If the dehydration is judged to be mild and the patient is conscious and cooperative, fluid should be given orally, but since old people rarely feel thirst it is essential that rehydration should be controlled by a nurse. An input chart should be kept and, if it is clear that there is difficulty in maintaining an intake of, say, 2 l a day, recourse should be made to intravenous therapy.

The impaired homeostasis which places old people at risk of dehydration, places them at extreme risk of developing fluid overload if they are given parenteral fluids. A reasonable regime is to start with between 2 and 3 l per day depending upon the level of the blood urea and the serum sodium. Serum sodium and blood urea levels should be checked daily, and once these show a substantial fall, the parenteral fluid intake should be reduced to about 2 l per day. If the patient begins to take fluids orally, this should be taken into account so that the total intake does not exceed 2 l. A reasonable balance of intravenous fluids is to give 500 ml of normal saline to 1 l to 5% dextrose. Potassium supplementation should be given if a low serum potassium concentration indicates this. More vigorous replacement is necessary if the dehydration is due to non-ketotic hyperglycaemia (Chap. 5). Plasma expanders may be indicated where there is hypotension particularly where this has been associated with protein loss or hypoalbuminaemia.

During this time, a close watch should be kept for signs of jugular venous congestion, tachycardia, peripheral or sacral oedema, and pulmonary oedema. Ideally, the central venous pressure should be monitored, but this should only be attempted if there are medical and nursing staff sufficiently experienced to service and monitor equipment. Measurement of the urinary volume and osmolality may give additional information in the effectiveness of fluid replacement, but difficulties in collecting this may make it impracticable.

Patients sometimes become dehydrated even although they are already receiving hospital care. This emphasises the importance of identifying patients at risk, and regularly monitoring their progress by estimation of blood urea and electrolytes. Nurses should also be advised to supervise and cajole such patients into increasing their fluid intake.

Hypernatraemia

As discussed above the vast majority of cases of hypernatraemia in elderly patients are associated with dehydration. The underlying cause in such patients is usually clear. Severe hypernatraemia may also occur in hyperosmolar non-ketotic diabetic coma (Chap. 4).

Occasionally, hypernatraemia is due to acquired diabetes insipidus. In old age, nephrogenic diabetes insipidus is usually secondary to chronic renal disease associated with tubular damage. It may be a feature of renal impairment associated with hypercalcaemia, hypokalaemia and toxicity from drugs including lithium, demeclocycline and amphotericin. Patients with nephropathy are dependent on intact thirst mechanisms to correct their dehydration. In elderly patients, these homeostatic mechanisms may be deranged. Thirst appreciation may also be compromised by hypothalamic damage or reduced consciousness.

Cranial diabetes is rare in an elderly patient but may complicate a head injury, while metastases in the hypothalamic area from carcinoma of bronchus or breast are also potential causes, as are large pituitary tumours and granulomatous lesions. In a proportion of cases no cause is found and hypothalamic vascular lesions may play a part.

Patients with diabetes insipidus usually complain of polyuria and thirst before hypernatraemia supervenes (sodium > 155 mmol/l). At this stage they may lapse into unconsciousness. As noted above, cranial diabetes insipidus may occur in an unconscious patient with a head injury; clearly this is a situation in which signs of hypernatraemia and dehydration should be sought.

Investigation

If the urine volume is less than 2.5 l per 24 h, then a patient does not have polyuria and diabetes insipidus is unlikely, unless there is intracranial disease with grossly defective thirst mechanisms. Demonstration of diabetes insipidus involves applying a stimulus to vasopressin (AVP) production. Traditionally, this is achieved by either water deprivation or a hypertonic saline infusion. Ideally, both tests should be accompanied by measurements of plasma AVP levels, but these are not widely available outside the research context. The hypertonic saline infusion test is contra-indicated in old age, but a water deprivation test may be undertaken if an elderly patient is otherwise fit and cooperative. A satisfactory protocol is discussed in Chap. 12. It must be emphasised that the patient must be weighed accurately and the test terminated if the weight falls by more than 5% of the initial weight. At the end of the test desmopressin (DDAVP) is administered to determine whether the renal tubules respond to AVP, thus to distinguish cranial from nephrogenic diabetes insipidus. Measurement of plama AVP concentrations facilitates the distinction between cranial and nephrogenic diabetes insipidus, in that patients with the latter have high plasma AVP concentrations.

If an elderly patient is unfit or insufficiently cooperative for fluid deprivation testing, then the effect of desmopressin on serum sodium and osmolality and urinary osmolality should be measured.

Management

Cranial diabetes insipidus is treated with desmopressin (DDAVP) intranasally, the usual dose being 10–20 µg twice daily. Use of this medication requires active cooperation and some dexterity on the part of the patient. It may also be administered parenterally, intramuscularly or intravenously, the usual dose being 1–4 µg and the duration of effect being 12–24 h.

Patients with partial cranial diabetes insipidus may respond to clofibrate or chlorpropamide. Both potentiate the action of endogenous AVP and clofibrate also stimulates AVP release. In non-diabetic individuals chlorpropamide sometimes induces hypoglycaemia.

Paradoxically, nephrogenic diabetes insipidus is managed with thiazide diuretics, e.g. bendrofluazide 5–10 mg daily. The mechanism of action is unclear but it may be that diuretic-induced sodium deficiency interferes with the ability of the kidney to excrete water. It should be noted that in cases of diabetes insipidus secondary to long-standing obstructive neuropathy release of the obstruction does not usually result in early cure of the AVP insensitivity.

Hyponatraemia

It is important to distinguish between patients presenting with chronic hyponatraemia and those presenting with hyponatraemia of recent onset since their aetiology, physiology, presentation and management are quite different.

Aetiology and Pathophysiology

Many old people admitted to hospital have a low serum sodium concentration. In a review of patients admitted to a geriatric assessment unit, 11.3% had a serum sodium concentration of less than 130 mmol/l, and 4.5% less than 125 mmol/l (Sunderam and Mankikar 1983). The prevalence of patients with a concentration of less than 125 mmol/l was lower in a series of patients admitted to a general medical unit (Kennedy et al. 1978).

Table 9.1 lists the causes of hyponatraemia identified in a few elderly patients admitted to the geriatric unit with hyponatraemia (Sunderam and Mankikar 1983). Diuretic treatment was by far the most common cause, but inappropriate

Table 9.1. Causes of hyponatraemia in elderly patients (Sunderam and Mankikar 1983)

Cause	Percentage proportion
Diuretics	64
Intravenous fluids	14
Inappropriate ADH secretion	18
"Sick cell" syndrome	9
Diabetes mellitus	5
Gastro-intestinal loss	4
Chronic liver disease	5

Note: Some patients suffered from more than one cause.

secretion of antidiuretic hormone (SIADH) and the "sick cell syndrome" were also common.

Hyponatraemia of acute onset is commonly seen in the post-operative situation when circulating concentrations of AVP are uniformly high. In elderly patients, this is particularly common after transuretheral prostatectomy where, in addition to the administration of intravenous fluids, bladder irrigation with large volumes of fluid exacerbates hyponatraemia. Dilution by the inappropriate use of fluid is also encountered in patients with burns or excessive electrolyte losses from the gastro-intestinal tract. Compulsive water drinking is another cause of acute hyponatraemia, although whether this is a problem with demented elderly patients remains to be documented.

On pathophysiological grounds, chronic hyponatraemia can be divided into four main types, based on the estimated extracellular fluid (ECF) volume and the urinary sodium excretion (Robinson 1985).

Type 1. The primary problem is that of dehydration; this is followed by water retention due to an increase in AVP release, which is not matched by a comparable degree of sodium conservation in the distal renal tubules. There is thus an imbalance between water and sodium retention so that the patient becomes hyponatraemic even although the urinary sodium concentration is low (<20 mmol/l). This may occur in patients in whom gastro-intestinal electrolyte loss is replaced with water, and in patients treated with excessive doses of diuretics.

Type 2. There is volume depletion with a continued high loss of sodium in the urine (>25 mmol/l). This can occur in both Addison's disease and in intrinsic renal disorders.

Type 3. There is over expansion of the ECF. Even although the urinary excretion of sodium is reduced (<20 mmol/l) this is not sufficient to prevent a dilution effect. This is a common feature in patients with cirrhosis, congestive heart failure or nephrotic syndrome where the total body sodium is increased, and there is an even greater increase in the ECF volume.

Type 4. The patient has a normal ECF volume but has an increased urinary sodium loss. This can occur in congestive cardiac failure where volume expansion provokes excessive atrial natriuretic peptide secretion. This results in a situation where the ECF volume returns to normal, but where there is excessive sodium loss with resultant hyponatraemia. This problem also arises where there is an inappropriate increase in the secretion of AVP [syndrome of inappropriate secretion of anti-diuretic hormone (SIADH)]. There are many potential causes of this in elderly patients (Table 9.2), the commonest being a chest infection. In many of these situations the mechanism of excessive AVP secretion is unclear, but it is thought that in chest infections, stimulation of AVP release via atrial volume receptors may be important. Again, a number of stresses including neurological insults can stimulate AVP secretion. In tumour-associated SIADH the tumour secretes AVP or AVP-like substances. Finally, a number of drugs including clofi-brate, chlorpropamide, and carbamazepine can stimulate AVP release or sensitise the kidney to the hormone.

Table 9.2. Causes of inappropriate secretion of anti-diuretic hormone

Malignant tumours – bronchus, prostate, thymus, pancreas
Neurological disorders – head injury, brain tumour, cerebrovascular accidents, meningitis, encephalitis
Lung infections – pneumonia, tuberculosis
Alcohol withdrawal
Hypothyroidism
Drugs

Presentation

The symptoms of acute and chronic hyponatraemia have been well reviewed (Arieff 1984). In the post-operative period, acute hyponatraemia usually occurs about 48 h after surgery, when there is confusion, and an altered level of consciousness which may progress to grand mal seizures (Arieff 1986). These clinical features are the result of cerebral oedema and brain swelling. The picture is different in chronic hyponatraemia, where solute is lost within the brain cells, so that cerebral oedema does not usually occur even when there are very low serum sodium levels. Accordingly, the symptoms associated with chronic hyponatraemia are non-specific and include weakness, confusion, ataxia and muscle twitching (Table 9.3). Some of these symptoms are so common in sick elderly patients that it is often difficult to establish a link with hyponatraemia in individual subjects. In cases of hyponatraemia where there is a decreased intravascular volume, there may be postural dizziness and hypotension.

Investigation

A clinical assessment including a history of drugs, and a thorough physical examination may clarify the cause of the hyponatraemia. This should be supplemented by a chest X-ray.

Assessment of serum electrolytes and osmolality and simultaneously urinary sodium and osmolality provides further useful information. In SIADH the serum sodium is often in the range 110–125 mmol/l with correspondingly low osmolality and the urinary osmolality is often around 500–600 mosmol/kg with the urinary

Table 9.3. Proportion of patients with serum sodium of 120 mmol/l or less with neurological symptoms (Daggett et al. 1982)

Abnormality	Percentage proportion with abnormality
Hemiparesis	3.3
Monoparesis	3.3
Rigidity	3.3
Extrapyramidal tremor	4.3
Cerebellar ataxia	6.6
Nystagmus	4.3
Pupillary irregularity	2.2
Convulsions	10.9

sodium greater than 40 mmol/l. If there is any possibility of a diagnosis of Addison's disease then a short Synacthen test (Chap. 11) is mandatory. Thyroid function tests are also of value in the investigation of unexplained hyponatraemia. Other investigations depend on the clinical features noted.

Management

The management of acute hyponatraemia depends firstly on its recognition, particularly as a cause of altered consciousness or seizures in the early post-operative period. Acute hyponatraemia has a mortality of around 50% in comparison to one of 12% in patients with long-standing hyponatraemia (Arieff et al. 1976). The evidence (which is largely anecdotal) favours rapid correction of acute hyponatraemia. The administration of normal or hypertonic saline reduces cerebral oedema, the main cause of altered consciousness, and seizures. In one recent study, a specially prepared solution of hypertonic saline was administered via a central line to five acutely hyponatraemic patients with seizures. Four made a full recovery with no neurological sequelae (Worthley and Thomas 1986). In another report, patients with acute hyponatraemia had this treated much more gradually until they recovered consciousness (Arieff 1986). Seven of these patients, however, went back into coma after 2–6 days and either died or remained in a permanent vegetative state.

From this information it would seem appropriate in acute hyponatraemia, with an altered consciousness level or seizures, that the serum sodium should be allowed to rise by approximately 2 mmol/l/h using hypertonic saline (3%) until the serum sodium is at a "safe" level (120–130 mmol/l). Thereafter, further correction is achieved by the normal homeostatic mechanism (Narins 1986). Acute correction of hyponatraemia can also be performed by infusing normal saline and injecting parenteral frusemide, which causes a relatively greater loss of water than sodium.

By contrast, there are considerable dangers in the rapid correction of the serum sodium concentration of chronically hyponatraemic patients. In one report, correction of the serum sodium concentration by more than 12 mmol/l over 24 h resulted in the severe neurological syndrome of central pontine (osmotic) myelinolysis (Sterns et al. 1986). A review of the literature established 13 cases of thiazide- or SIADH-induced hyponatraemia where gentle correction of the condition resulted in uneventful recovery (Sterns et al. 1986). It appears, therefore, that chronically hyponatraemic patients should not be aggressively treated but that, if diuretics are the cause, these should be discontinued and fluid restricted to 800 ml per day.

If chronic hyponatraemia is due to SIADH and cure of the primary pathology is not possible, fluid restriction should be the first line of management but may need to be supplemented by the use of the antibiotic demeclocycline (De Troyer and Demanet 1975). This causes a functional nephrogenic diabetes insipidus with increased water loss and correction of the hyponatraemia. The usual dose range is 600–1200 mg daily, titrated according to its effect on the serum sodium level. An alternative, but more toxic drug in this situation is lithium. In other situations, specific causes of hyponatraemia should receive appropriate treatment. Examples are the use of mineralocorticoids in Addison's disease, and the use of ACE inhibitors in severe congestive heart failure.

Hypokalaemia

Aetiology

There is a decline in total body potassium levels with increasing age in both men and women (Edmonds et al. 1975). Most of this is the result of a decline in fat-free mass, but there also may be a slight decrease in the intracellular concentration of potassium (MacLennan et al. 1977). This, in turn, is probably a manifestation of decreased physical activity in old age. Certainly, in younger age groups, habitual exercise has an important effect on total body potassium levels (Burkinshaw et al. 1971).

Some old people have very low intakes of potassium, but there is considerable geographical variation in this (MacLennan 1987). Mental and ill health may affect intakes, but this is not universal and in some hospital groups potassium intakes are very high (MacLennan et al. 1975).

Studies in the 1960s and early 1970s suggested that congestive cardiac failure might be a cause of potassium depletion. However, there were limitations in their measurement techniques and more recent surveys suggest that there is only minimal potassium depletion even in elderly people with cardiac failure (Ibrahim et al. 1978; Lye 1982).

Though ageing, nutritional deficiency, and cardiac failure may effect total body potassium status, they rarely affect serum concentrations and in old age the most common cause of a low serum potassium concentration is diuretic therapy.

Treatment with a thiazide diuretic produces a striking reduction in serum levels which is sustained for at least a year after the start of treatment (Wilkinson et al. 1975). Loop diuretics produce a smaller but nonetheless significant drop in serum levels (Morgan and Davidson 1980). In contrast to their effect on serum levels, diuretics produce little or no change in total body potassium levels (Wilkinson et al. 1975). The relevance of these findings depends upon whether or not it is the absolute potassium level or the ratio of intra- to extracellular potassium which is responsible for clinical signs. Debate continues on this issue (Steiness 1981).

The other common cause of hypokalaemia is fluid loss from the gastro-intestinal tract and in an elderly patient it is important to consider the possibility of chronic laxative or liquorice abuse or, rarely, a villous adenoma of the rectum. Primary hyperaldosteronism or Cushing's syndrome due to ectopic ACTH secretion by a tumour may also cause hypokalaemia.

Presentation

Hypokalaemia is associated with a change in the resting membrane potential of the myocardium, and this has a serious effect on cardiac irritability and conduction (Haddy 1973). Electrocardiographic manifestations include ST sagging, T wave inversion and a prominent U wave (Fig. 9.1). In old age, these changes are often masked by myocardial ischaemia or drug therapy.

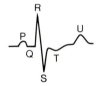

Fig. 9.1. Electrocardiographic changes in hypokalaemia.

Clinical manifestations of depletion include first- and second-degree heart block, supraventricular and ventricular extrasystoles, atrial fibrillation or flutter, atrial or ventricular tachycardia and ventricular fibrillation (Hollifield and Slaton 1981). Fortunately, the more serious arrhythmias are rare, but their risk is greatly enhanced if the patient is also being given a cardiac glycoside (Steiness 1981).

Severe hypokalaemia can give rise to profound muscle weakness. An extreme example of this is hypokalaemic periodic paralysis, occasionally identified in young adults (Ward 1978). There are occasional instances of drug-induced severe hypokalaemia producing similar problems in the elderly. It is much more doubtful whether chronic potassium depletion due to a reduced intake is an important cause of muscle weakness. Early reports of a reduced grip strength in depleted elderly patients, corrected by potassium supplements, have not been confirmed (Burr et al. 1975).

There has been speculation that potassium depletion might be responsible for mental impairment and depression in malnourished old people. In one study, treatment with potassium supplements achieved an improvement in cognitive function and in a depression rating (Judge 1972). The findings have not been substantiated, however. Another group of elderly patients with depression had low total exchangeable potassium levels, but the depletion could be explained as the result of increased adrenocortical activity associated with stress (Cox and Orme 1973). In the same investigation, patients with dementia had reduced potassium levels, but this was a reflection of a decreased skeletal muscle rather than a true deficiency.

A final intriguing possibility is that hypokalaemia interferes with pancreatic beta cell function, and thus decreases insulin synthesis and secretion (Helderman et al. 1983). This may be the indirect route whereby thiazide diuretics are associated with impaired carbohydrate tolerance.

Prevention and Treatment

Since only a minority of patients on diuretics develop clinically significant hypokalaemia, there is debate as to whether all patients on diuretics should receive potassium supplements or potassium sparing agents. A reasonable compromise is to monitor electrolyte levels for the first 2 months of treatment, and only intervene in patients with a serum potassium concentration of less than 3.0 mmol/l or in those also receiving digoxin.

Prevention of hypokalaemia requires a dose of at least 24 mmol of potassium per day. Even on this, a proportion of sick elderly patients remain hypokalaemic, and require as much as 60 mmol per day to achieve normal status (Lye 1980). In practical terms, this means that even if elderly patients are on potassium supplements, their serum levels should be monitored for at least 2 months, and that while a starting dose of 24 mmol per day is reasonable, a proportion will require to have this increased to 60 mmol. The quantity of potassium in preparations containing a diuretic with potassium supplements is generally too small to be of value.

An alternative is to use a potassium-sparing agent, and there are a variety of formulations which combine a diuretic with one of these (Table 9.4). All such preparations reduce but do not eliminate the incidence of diuretic-induced hypokalaemia, so that patients treated in this way should have their serum electrolyte levels monitored for the first few weeks. There is also the risk with these combined preparations of increasing the urinary excretion of sodium and causing hyponatraemia, hyporolaemia and dehydration.

Table 9.4. Diuretics combined with potassium-sparing agents

Formulation	Thiazide	Potassium sparer
Aldactide 50	Hydroflumethiazide 50 mg	Spironolactone 50 mg
Dyazide	Hydrochlorothiazide 25 mg	Triamterene 50 mg
Moduretic	Hydrochlorothiazide 50 mg	Amiloride 5 mg
Frumil	Frusemide 40 mg	Amiloride 5 mg
Frusene	Frusemide 40 mg	Triamterene 50 mg
Lasilactone	Frusemide 20 mg	Spironolactone 50 mg

Hyperkalaemia

This usually refers to a serum potassium value of more than 5.5 mmol/l. One of the results of vigorous treatment and prevention of hypokalaemia in old people is that a proportion develop hyperkalaemia. The prevalence of this ranges between that of 3.4% for patients on frusemide and potassium supplements, to one of 12% for those on a combination of hydrochlorothiazide and triamterene (Dyazide) (Bender et al. 1967; Lawson 1974). Since there is no simple way of predicting which patient will become hyperkalaemic, the only way of tackling the problem is to monitor serum electrolyte levels until these have become stabilised. Since the distal tubule of the kidney is a major site for potassium homeostasis, patients with impaired renal function may be at particular risk of developing hyperkalaemia on a combined diuretic and potassium conserving agent.

Though the inappropriate use of potassium supplements or sparing agents is by far the most common cause for hyperkalaemia in old age, other factors should be considered (Table 9.5). An illustration is that in one series, an 80-year-old woman with hyporeninaemic hypoaldosteronism (a complication of long-standing diabetes mellitus) and a 73-year-old woman with indomethacin-induced hyperkalaemia were identified (Walmsley et al. 1984). More common causes include diabetic ketoacidosis, and acute or chronic renal failure.

Table 9.5. Causes of hyperkalaemia

Extrarenal
Oral or intravenous supplements
Burns
Crush injury
Reperfusion of ischaemic tissue
Diabetic ketoacidosis
Digoxin toxicity

Renal
Acute and chronic renal failure
Drugs
(a) potassium sparing agents
(b) prostaglandin inhibitors, e.g. indomethacin,
    ibuprofen
(c) ACE inhibitors

Adrenal disorders (see Chap. 8)
Addison's disease

Presentation

The problem of hyperkalaemia in the elderly has received little attention in the recent literature. Its signs and symptoms resemble those of hypokalaemia and include muscle weakness, cardiac arrhythmias and varying degrees of heart block. If the serum level exceeds 7.5 mmol/l, the risk of cardiac arrest is high. Typical electrocardiographic features of hyperkalaemia include low amplitude P waves, widening of the QRS complex, prolongation of the QT interval, increased amplitude of T waves and depression of the ST segment (Fig. 9.2).

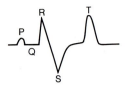

Fig. 9.2. Electrocardiographic changes in hyperkalaemia.

Treatment

This is often required as an emergency measure and should be as for younger patients using an insulin and dextrose infusion in the acute state.

Hypomagnesaemia

There is little definitive information on magnesium status in the elderly. However, compared with young adults, old people have a relatively low intake of magnesium (MacLennan, unpublished) (Table 9.6).

Table 9.6. Intake of magnesium (mean ± 2 standard deviations) in elderly patients attending a day hospital (MacLennan, personal observation)

Sex	Age	Number	Intake (mmol/day)
M	65–74	6	64 ± 26
M	75+	9	72 ± 13
F	65–74	5	41 ± 18
F	75+	27	63 ± 25

Patients on diuretics are further compromised by increased magnesium loss and, since the main site of magnesium reabsorption is the ascending limb of the loop of Henle, loop diuretics such as frusemide or bumetanide, can cause particularly severe depletion (Ryan et al. 1984). However, since 5% of magnesium is reabsorbed from the distal tubule, thiazide diuretics have a similar if less striking effect on magnesium status. Magnesium deficiency may also occur in patients with severe gastro-intestinal fluid loss.

The diagnosis of hypomagnesaemia is normally made on the basis of a low serum magnesium concentration. This probably provides an underestimate of the extent of the problem, and recently developed techniques for measuring intralymphocyte concentrations may throw further light on the problem (Ryan et al. 1981).

Presentation

Hypomagnesaemia has a serious effect on cardiac function (Sheehan and White 1982). Electrocardiographic changes are dependent on whether or not there is also hypokalaemia or hypocalcaemia but they include peaked P waves, U waves and low voltage QRS complexes and T waves (Fig. 9.3). Other manifestations include a reversible atrial fibrillation and increased sensitivity to the cardiotoxic effects of cardiac glycosides. There also is circumstantial evidence that chronic magnesium depletion, in areas where there is "soft" drinking water, is responsible for an increased incidence of arrythmias causing sudden death.

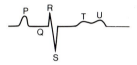

Fig. 9.3. Electrocardiographic changes in hypomagnesaemia.

Experimental magnesium depletion in human volunteers has resulted in muscle weakness, fasciculation and tetany, but there is no evidence as yet that magnesium depletion is an important cause of muscle weakness in the elderly or that this can be corrected by supplements (Cronin and Knochel 1983). Less specific effects include tremor, ataxia, apathy and depression, but these features are so common in sick old people that any relationship to magnesium deficiency would be hard to prove.

Hypomagnesaemia is often associated with both hypocalcaemia and hypokalaemia (Cronin and Knochel 1983). The former is due to the influx of calcium from the extra- to the intracellular compartment and also to reduced secretion of parathyroid hormone in hypomagnesaemia. If the condition is misdiagnosed as primary hypocalcaemia and calcium supplements given, symptoms of hypomagnesia are accentuated (Leading Article 1976). Extra- and intracellular concentrations of magnesium and potassium seem to be closely linked with one another so that a change in one is invariably followed by a change in the other. This means that a low potassium level associated with magnesium depletion is very resistant to treatment with potassium supplements.

At present the relevance of magnesium depletion to disability in old age is speculative, and definitive research is badly needed.

Treatment

Correction of depletion with oral magnesium is limited by the problem that most preparations act as osmostic laxatives and cause troublesome diarrhoea. Fortunately, most potassium-sparing agents also have a magnesium-sparing effect so that treatment with amiloride, spironolactone or triamterene is usually effective (Dyckner and Wester 1984). In severe depletion it may be necessary to give an intravenous infusion of between 8 and 12 g of magnesium sulphate.

References

Arieff AI (1984) Central nervous system manifestations of disordered sodium metabolism. Clin Endocrinol Metab 13: 269–294

Arieff AI (1986) Hyponatraemia convulsions respiratory arrest and permanent brain damage after elective surgery in healthy women. N Engl J Med 314: 1529–1535

Arieff AI, Llach F, Massry SG (1976) Neurological manifestations and morbidity of hyponatraemia: correlation with brain and water electrolytes. Medicine 55: 121–129

Bender AD, Carter Cl, Hansen KB (1967) Use of diuretic combination of triamterene and hydrochlorothiazide in elderly patients. J Am Geriatr Soc 15: 166–173

Burkinshaw L, Cotes JE, Jones PRM, Kribbs AV (1971) Prediction of total body potassium from anthropometric measurements. Hum Biol 43: 344–355

Burr ML, St Leger AS, Westlake CA, Davies HEF (1975) Dietary potassium deficiency in the elderly: a controlled trial. Age Ageing 5: 148–151

Cox JR, Orme JE (1973) Body water, electrolyte and psychological test performances in elderly patients. Gerontol Clin 15: 203–208

Cronin RE, Knochel JP (1983) Magnesium deficiency. Adv Intern Med 28: 509–533

Daggett P, Deanfield J, Moss F (1982) Neurological aspects of hyponatraemia. Postgrad Med J 58: 737–740

De Troyer A, Demanet JC (1975) Correction of anti-diuresis by demeclocycline. N Engl J Med 293: 915–918

Dyckner T, Wester PO (1984) Intracellular magnesium loss after diuretic administration. Drugs 28: (Suppl 1): 161–166

Edmonds CJ, Jasani BM, Smith T (1975) Total body potassium and body fat estimation in relationship to height, sex, age, malnutrition and obesity. Clin Sci Mol Med 48: 431–440

Haddy FJ (1973) Potassium deficiency and heart function. J Chronic Dis 26: 467–469

Helderman JH, Elahi D, Anderson DK et al. (1983) Prevention of the glucose intolerance of thiazide diuretics by maintenance of body potassium. Diabetes 32: 106–111

Hollifield JW, Slaton PE (1981) Thiazide diuretics, hypokaleamia and cardiac arrythmias. Acta Med Scand [Suppl] 647: 67–73

Ibrahim IK, Ritch AES, MacLennan WJ, May T (1978) Are potassium supplements for the elderly necessary? Age Ageing 7: 165–170

Judge TG (1972) Potassium metabolism in the elderly. In: Carlson LA (ed) Nutrition in old age. Almquist and Wiksell, Stockholm, pp 86–89

Kennedy PGE, Mitchell DM, Hoffbrand BI (1978) Severe hyponatraemia in hospital inpatients. Br Med J 2: 1251–1253

Lawson DH (1974) Adverse reactions to potassium chloride. Q J Med 43, 433–440

Leading Article (1976) Magnesium deficiency. Lancet 1: 523–524

Leaf A (1984) Dehydration in the elderly. N Engl J Med 311: 791–792

Lye M (1980) Potassium supplements in elderly patients with cardiac failure. Practitioner 224: 1314 1315

Lye M (1982) Body potassium content and capacity of elderly individuals with and without cardiac failure. Cardiovasc Res 16: 22–25

MacLennan WJ (1987) Diuretic therapy and potassium balance. In: Swift CG (ed) Clinical pharmacology in the elderly. Marcel Dekker, New York, pp 179–212

MacLennan WJ, Lye MDW, May T (1977) The effect of potassium supplements on total body potassium levels in the elderly. Age Ageing 6: 46–50

MacLennan WJ, Martin P, Mason BJ (1975) Causes for reduced dietary intake in a long-stay care hospital. Age Ageing 4: 175–180

Morgan DB, Davidson C (1980) Hypokalaemia and diuretics: an analysis of publications. Br Med J 280: 905–908

Narins RG (1986) Therapy of hyponatraemia: does haste make waste: N Engl J Med 341: 1573–1575

Robinson AG (1985) Antidiuretic hormone secretion. Clin Endocrinol Metab 14: 55–88

Ryan MP, Ryan MF, Counihan TB (1981) The effects of diuretics on lymphocyte magnesium and potassium. Acta Med Scand [Suppl] 647: 153–161

Ryan MP, Devane J, Ryan MF, Counihan TB (1984) Effects of diuretics on the renal handling of magnesium. Drugs 28 (Suppl 1): 167–181

Sheehan J, White A (1982) Diuretic-associated hypokalaemia. Br Med J 285: 1157–1159

Steiness E (1981) Diuretics digitalis and arrythmias. Acta Med Scand [Suppl] 647: 75–78

Sterns RM, Riggs JE, Schochet SS (1986) Osmotic demyelination syndrome following correction of hyponatremia. N Engl J Med, 314: 1535–1542

Sunderam SG, Mankikar GD (1983) Hyponatraemia in the elderly. Age Ageing 12: 77–80

Walmsley RN, White GH, Cain M et al. (1984) Hyperkalaemia in the elderly. Clin Chem 30: 1409–1412

Ward D (1978) Hypokalaemic paralysis. Br Med J 2: 93–94

Wilkinson PR, Hesp R, Issler H, Raftery EB (1975) Total body and serum potassium during prolonged thiazide therapy for essential hypertension. Lancet 1: 759–762

Worthley WF, Thomas PD (1986) Treatment of hyponatraemic seizures with intravenous 29.2% saline. Br Med J 292: 168–170

10 Body Build and Nutritional Balance

In old age, a complex interaction between neuromuscular degeneration, physical activity, nutrient intake, metabolic activity and disease produces a wide range of changes in body build. At the one extreme there is the tiny emaciated bird-like lady of 95 who remains mentally and physically active, and at the other there is the 130 kg woman of 70 who has had three strokes, is chair-fast and imposes a major burden on relatives and nursing staff.

The management of both emaciation and obesity in old age is rarely straight-forward. A first step in this is an accurate clinical evaluation of the particular physiological, nutritional and pathological factors involved in an individual patient.

Age Changes in Body Build

Fat-Free Mass

There is a decline in fat-free mass throughout adult life (Fig. 10.1) (Novak 1972). Part of this is related to a decline in bone mass, but most is the result of a reduction in the quantity of skeletal muscle.

The principal explanation for this is that there is a loss of anterior horn neurones associated with denervation atrophy of skeletal muscle fibres (Fig. 10.2) (Tomlinson and Irving 1977). There is little neuronal loss under the age of 60, but thereafter there is an accelerated decline. Surviving neurones compensate for the denervation by developing axon branches to renervate denervated motor end plates. Eventually, however, neuronal loss is in excess of the capacity of the surviving neurones to reinnervate.

Muscle bulk is also influenced by physical activity. In one study there was a dramatic decline in the thigh muscle mass of steel workers in the year after their retirement (Fentem et al. 1976). Conversely, training programmes have increased the lean body mass of elderly men and women (Shephard 1978). Although old

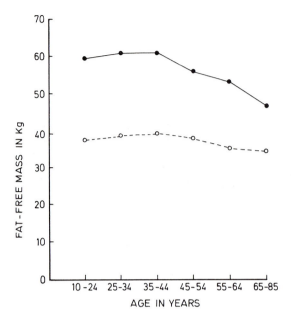

Fig. 10.1. Fat-free mass related to age in men (*solid circles*) and women (*open circles*). (After Novak, 1972.)

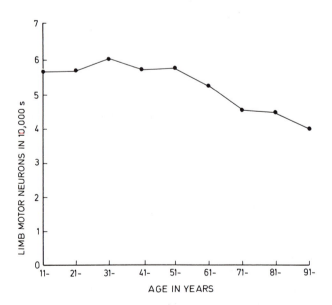

Fig. 10.2. Number of anterior horn neurones related to age. (After Tomlinson and Irving 1977.)

people have a reduced protein intake there is no evidence that, in good health, this has a significant effect on muscle mass.

Fat Mass

In healthy old people there is an increase in both absolute and percentage body fat (Novak 1972) (Fig. 10.3). It should be re-emphasised, however, that these observations relate to average changes and that there is a great deal of individual variation. Thus, there is little change in the fat mass of old people living in areas of the world with a limited food supply, or in elderly athletes (Shephard 1978). As yet, there is no evidence that changes in endocrine function are responsible for an increased fat mass in healthy old people.

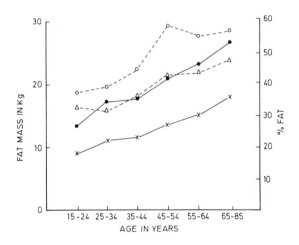

Fig. 10.3. Fat mass (*solid circles*, men; *open circles*, women) and percentage body fat (*crosses*, men; *triangles*, women) related to age. (After Novak 1972.)

Nutrient Intake

Amongst elderly people in the community there is a decline in the intake of most nutrients with increasing age (Table 10.1) (Lonergan et al. 1975). This change is a reflection of the total amount of food eaten. When nutrient intake is related to that for calories there is no evidence, with the possible exception of ascorbic acid in men, of a deterioration in the quality of diets with increasing age (Table 10.2).

Table 10.1. Daily nutrient intake related to age (Lonergan et al. 1975)

Nutrient	Daily intake in men aged		Daily intake in women aged	
	62–74	75–90	62–74	75–90
Energy (MJ)	10.5	9.1	7.4	6.9
Protein (g)	74.5	69.5	57.8	54.5
Calcium (mg)	958	964	799	786
Iron (mg)	11.7	10.7	9.0	8.1
Thiamine (mg)	0.9	0.9	0.8	0.7
Ascorbic acid (mg)	32.5	14.7	32.3	29.4
Vitamin D (µg)	3.1	2.6	2.0	1.8

Table 10.2. Nutrient intake per MJ related to age (using figures of Lonergan et al. 1975)

Nutrient per MJ	Daily intake in men aged		Daily intake in women aged	
	62–74	75–90	62–74	75–90
Protein (g)	7.1	7.6	7.8	7.9
Calcium (mg)	91	106	108	114
Iron (mg)	1.1	1.2	1.2	1.2
Thiamine (mg)	0.09	0.10	0.11	0.10
Ascorbic acid (mg)	3.1	1.6	4.4	4.3
Vitamin D (µg)	0.30	0.29	0.27	0.26

Gastro-intestinal Absorption

Ageing has a minor effect on both carbohydrate and fat absorption in the elderly (Webster and Leeming, 1975; Webster et al. 1977). These changes are of insufficient magnitude for them to be of practical importance in energy balance for the elderly.

Energy Expenditure

If account is taken of alterations in body composition, ageing has no effect on the basal metabolic rate of humans (Shock 1955). The apparent reduction in this is related to a decline of fat-free mass in old age.

It is more difficult to generalise on levels of physical activity in the elderly since this is influenced by a wide range of social, cultural and psychological, as well as physical factors (Shephard 1978). Retirement has a major effect on energy expenditure in men, and both sexes spend much less time actively involved in sports as they age. There are many exceptions to those trends, however, and some elderly farmers and forestry workers have an exceptionally high energy expenditure.

The only limiting factor to energy expenditure in fit elderly people is that ageing is associated with a decline in maximal exercise capacity measured as maximal oxygen uptake. In many situations, however, elderly people rarely exercise them-selves to this level, so it does not impose an important limitation on their daily activity (Sidney and Shephard 1977).

Nitrogen Balance

Nitrogen balance studies suggest that in healthy old people, protein requirements do not decline and may actually increase. Cheng et al. (1978) found that both young and old people required a protein intake of between 0.4 and 0.8 g/kg body weight to achieve a positive nitrogen balance. A more recent study suggested that protein requirements for old people may be substantially higher at 0.97 g/kg per day in negative nitrogen balance. These compare with intakes recommended by the Food and Agriculture Organisation of the World Health Organisation of 0.55 g/kg body weight for men and 0.42 g/kg body weight for women.

The mean intakes of protein in elderly men and women in the community are around double that recommended by the WHO (Table 10.3), (Lonergan et al. 1975). However, if the conclusions from nitrogen balance studies are correct, most old people have protein intakes which are only marginally in excess of their requirements and are thus at major risk if any stress is placed on their nitrogen balance.

Table 10.3. Mean intakes of protein in men and women over 62 (from Lonergan et al. 1975)

Sex	Age (years)	Mean intake (g per kg body weight)	Standard deviation
Male	62–74	1.09	0.24
	75–90	1.00	0.25
Female	62–74	0.92	0.18
	75–90	0.94	0.21

Nutrient Intake and Lifespan

Many laboratory studies have established that dietary restriction increases the lifespan of mice and rats (Masoro 1984). Additional features are that the physiological changes of ageing are delayed and the incidence of age-related dis-eases is reduced.

It would appear that the most important component of dietary restriction is calorie restriction. A reduction in protein intake alone has only a marginal effect on longevity. A further point is that there is an extension of maximum as well as median lifespan. This contrasts with observations in human populations where an improvement in the environment increases median survival, but has no effect on maximum span. The timing has been the subject of controversy. Initial studies suggested restriction in early life had a much greater effect on lifespan than that imposed later on. Several subsequent studies failed to confirm this.

Dietary restriction may delay ageing through a variety of physiological mechanisms. One is that it both delays and reduces an increase in serum cholesterol concentrations with age. There also are delays in the decline of immunological function and numbers of dopamine receptors. Age-related diseases delayed in rats include nephropathy and cardiomyopathy.

It has been suggested that dietary restriction increases lifespan by delaying maturation. However, since it is now clear that restriction after maturity also increases lifespan, this seems unlikely. Again, there is little to support the view that longevity is increased by prolonging the duration of growth. A more attractive explanation, that longevity is the result of a reduced incidence of obesity, was discarded when it emerged that there was no correlation between body fat and lifespan. Finally, there is increasing doubt that food restriction prolongs life by reducing the basal metabolic rate. At present, therefore, the precise mode of action of dietary restriction on ageing in laboratory animals is unclear.

Caution should be exercised when relating laboratory studies in rats to the human situation. One problem is that laboratory animals receive little exercise and have usually been overfed to ensure maximum growth. However, a recent report suggests that even if rats are allowed to choose their diets, those selecting a low intake have greater longevity (Ross et al. 1985).

Even if further evidence is adduced that dietary restriction is useful, it is difficult to see how its benefits can be investigated in man. Longitudinal studies would be too long to be practicable. Again, most populations with a low nutrient intake suffer from so many hostile environmental factors that any benefit from their dietary habits would be cancelled out. Finally, it would be impossible to collect accurate retrospective information on the earlier dietary intakes of an ageing population, and information on current intake might bear little relationship to past intake.

Reduced Weight and Muscle Wasting

Few old people who are otherwise healthy suffer from subnutrition and the problem occurs mainly in those with physical and mental incapacity. Thus, in a recent review, body weight, muscle mass and body fat were substantially higher in healthy old people than those attending a day centre or geriatric day hospital, or admitted to a psychogeriatric unit (Morgan et al. 1986) (Fig. 10.4).

Evaluation

Body build can be evaluated by relating total weight to the square of height, but this index is invalid in elderly patients with kyphosis or a lower-limb deformity. In clinical practice the simplest method of assessing fat mass is to measure the skinfold thickness over the triceps (TSF) of the non-dominant arm (MacLennan

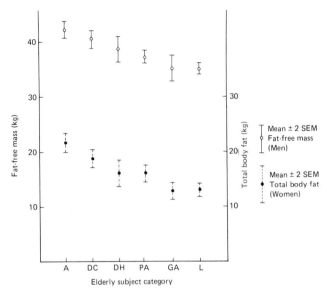

Fig. 10.4. Body build of subjects in different care groups. A: active and healthy; DC: day care; DH: day hospital; PA: psychogeriatric assessment unit; GA: geriatric assessment unit; L: long-stay care. (After Morgan et al. 1986.)

1985). A range of standard values for triceps thickness in old people living at home is now available (Burr and Phillips 1984).

Information on muscle mass can be obtained by also measuring the circumference of the arm at its mid-point (mid-arm circumference, MAC). This is used to estimate the arm muscle circumference (AMC) with the formula:

$$AMC \, (mm) = MAC \, (mm) - \pi \times TSF \, (mm)$$

Another index, arm muscle area (AMA) can be calculated from the formula:

$$AMA \, (mm^2) = \frac{AMC^2}{4\pi}$$

Standard values are also available for these indices (Burr and Phillips 1984).

The calculation of arm muscle area (AMA) has been further refined by using a correction factor to eliminate the effect of bone. Thus, corrected arm muscle area CAMA (cm^2) = AMC (cm^2) − 10 (males); CAMA (cm^2) = AMA (cm^2) −6.5 (females).

Studies on sick elderly patients suggest CAMA values of less than 16.0 cm^2 for men and 16.90 cm^2 for women over 65 are indicative of protein imbalance (Friedman et al. 1985a).

More accurate information on fat mass and fat-free mass can be obtained by estimating skinfold thicknesses over the triceps, biceps, subscapular and suprailiac areas. Tables are available which relate the sums of these values to fat mass and fat-free mass (Durnin and Womersley 1974). A caveat is that these tables have only been validated against body density up to the age of 72, so that their use in older subjects may provide misleading information.

Body composition can also be evaluated by using computerised tomography, or estimating the total body potassium or nitrogen. These techniques are time-consuming, involving expensive equipment which is not routinely available, and are only of value in research.

A large range of laboratory indices have been used to assess nutritional status. The most useful are the serum pre-albumin and albumin concentrations (Morgan et al. 1986). These, however, are not merely affected by protein intake. Hepatic protein synthesis, tissue breakdown, capillary permeability, and leakage from the gut or kidneys are also of major importance.

There is extensive information on vitamin status in the elderly (Kemm 1985). It is clear from this that such a wide range of factors affects circulating levels and there is such a large overlap of levels between malnourished patients and controls that assays are of limited value in the routine management of clinical problems in the elderly.

Aetiology

The causes of weight loss and muscle wasting in old age vary with the population studied. In patients with relatively stable conditions in long-stay geriatric units, there is a reasonable correlation between protein intake and muscle mass, and serum prealbumin and albumin levels (MacLennan et al. 1977; Morgan et al. 1986). This suggests that dietary deficiency is an important cause of muscle wasting and hypoalbuminaemia in many frail old people. The relationship between energy intake and skinfold thickness is either absent or minimal (MacLennan et al. 1975; Morgan et al. 1986). Factors other than dietary intake would thus appear to have a major influence on fat mass in old age.

While age itself has relatively little effect on gastro-intestinal function, malabsorption is relatively common in frail elderly patients, particularly those with signs of gross nutritional deficiency such as iron deficiency anaemia or osteomalacia (Montgomery et al. 1978). More common causes of malabsorption in this group are previously undiagnosed coeliac disease, pancreatic insufficiency, previous partial gastrectomy and jejunal diverticular disease (Price et al. 1973) (Table 10.4). Since the characteristics of elderly patients, from whom those with malabsorption have been selected, have not been defined, there is no firm information on the prevalence of malabsorption in the elderly, or its absolute importance as a cause of muscle wasting or weight loss.

In many old people a major factor in weight loss and tissue destruction is an increase in energy expenditure and protein breakdown. Thus, in one review of long-stay patients, the skinfold thicknesses of those with disorders associated with increased energy expenditure such as thyrotoxicosis, malignancy or chronic sepsis were much lower than in the remainder of the group (MacLennan et al. 1975). Again, amongst patients admitted to a geriatric assessment unit, a far higher proportion of patients with hypoalbuminaemia suffered from an acute illness than the

Table 10.4. Causes of steatorrhoea in patients aged 50 years and over (Price et al. 1977)

Coeliac disease	16
Carcinoma of pancreas	4
Other pancreatic disease	10
Partial gastrectomy	8
Jejunal diverticula	2
Tropical sprue	2
Diabetes mellitus	1
Scleroderma	1
Whipple's disease	1
Undetermined	1

remainder with a normal serum albumin concentration (Friedman et al. 1985b). In this study there was no relationship between hypoalbuminaemia and muscle wasting, but this could be explained by the fact that the acute illness had not persisted for long enough for a negative nitrogen balance to have an effect on the latter. Certainly, in most patients, there is a strong association between either injury or acute or chronic illness and muscle wasting (Rennie and Harrison 1984). Although patients with these disorders are often in negative nitrogen balance, this is largely a result of increased breakdown of protein in the viscera. In skeletal muscle the primary defect is that of impaired protein synthesis. Since the rate of breakdown in skeletal muscle is unchanged, the net consequence is that of muscle wasting.

Treatment

The theoretical solution to weight loss and muscle wasting would be to increase energy and protein intake. Practical problems are that sick old people have poor appetites, and that high concentrations of protein may cause diarrhoea. Although a skilled dietician may be able to devise meals which are both palatable and protein rich, these are often unsuccessful and recourse may have to be made to enteral feeding through a fine-bore nasogastric tube.

This approach has been used successfully in elderly patients recovering from a factured proximal femur (Bastow et al. 1983). The regimen chosen was to supplement the normal diet of patients with 1 l per day of Clinifeed Iso containing 4.2 MJ energy and 28 g protein. This was delivered over 8 h overnight through a fine-bore nasogastric tube attached to a peristaltic pump. There are many other clinical situations in the elderly where enteral feeding might be useful, but little information has been published on this as yet.

Obesity

While an increased fat mass is not an inevitable concomitant of ageing, obesity has become an increasing problem amongst elderly men and women in industrial countries. Apart from its association with a wide range of disease, severe obesity has serious effects on the mobility of old people with neurological and locomotor disorders. As such it is a major cause of incapacity in old age.

Aetiology

Intake and Energy Expenditure

The energy intake of obese elderly patients is no greater than that of those with a normal or reduced fat mass (MacLennan et al. 1975). It follows, therefore, that there must be differences in the energy expenditure of lean and obese subjects. If the resting metabolic rate (RMR) alone is measured this actually increases with fat mass (Garrow and Webster 1985). When the ratio of RMR to fat mass is estimated, however, this remains constant throughout the range of fat mass. This suggests that the RMR of pre-obese patients, though not reduced, is certainly not increased.

The energy expenditure (thermic effect) of digesting food is also similar in lean and obese subjects (Segal and Gatton 1983). Exercise, however, potentiates the thermic effect of food, and when this was investigated in thin and obese individuals it was increased by 2.54 times in the former, but only by 1.01 times in the latter. As with the RMR, the energy expenditure for a standard work load is increased in obese people, but is no different from that of lean subjects if expressed as a ratio of body surface area.

Further studies are required to validate these findings. They illustrate, however, that differences in energy expenditure between thin and obese people may be subtle and not identified by standard oxygen consumption tests. It might be argued that such subtle differences might be so marginal as to be of little practical importance. However, a marginal imbalance over many years would be sufficient to result in a gradual but substantial weight gain.

A further issue is whether disability associated with immobility and reduced energy expenditure is an important cause of obesity in elderly invalids. Most studies suggest that the energy intakes of disabled elderly patients are substantially lower than those of healthy old people (MacLennan 1983). It remains to be established whether the decline in expenditure exceeds that of intake, or whether the former exceeds the latter. A further complication is that many of the illnesses responsible for disability such as rheumatoid arthritis, congestive cardiac failure or malignancy may cause stress and thus increase the resting metabolic rate.

Endocrine Function

Abnormalities of endocrine function are demonstrable in obesity, but these are probably the result rather than the cause of the condition (Jung 1984). One attractive hypothesis is that weight gain is the result of the increase in cortisol synthesis and utilisation found in obese people. However, these metabolic changes can be reduced by dieting. They can also be induced by increasing the food intakes of lean volunteers.

Obese patients also exhibit a receptor, and, in severe obesity, post-receptor resistance to insulin (Chap. 4). Dieting, however, increases both the number of insulin receptors and the tissue sensitivity to insulin.

Changes in anterior pituitary function reflected in an impaired growth hormone and prolactin secretion are another characteristic of obesity. Even after weight reduction growth hormone and prolactin secretion remain reduced (Jung et al. 1982). Since noradrenaline secretion is also reduced, it seems likely that the changes are the result of an alteration in hypothalamic function. Whether these are the cause or the effect of obesity requires further investigation, and whether these endocrine abnormalities persist in the obese elderly remains unclear.

Complications

Locomotor

In terms of its immediate effect upon the mobility and self-care capacity of elderly individuals, the most important complication of obesity in the elderly is osteo-arthritis. There is a particularly strong association between obesity and arthritis of the weight-bearing joints in women (Leach et al. 1973) (Table 10.5). It is unclear whether obesity initiates or merely exacerbates the symptoms of coexistent disease.

Table 10.5. Proportion of patients with osteoarthritis of the knees with obesity (Leach et al. 1973)

	Percentage prevalence of obesity	
	Men	Women
Osteoarthritis	35	83
Controls	38	42

Excess weight also imposes a strain on the feet (Munsey 1981). In particular there is excessive pronation of the medical longitudinal arch leading to strain on the legs and back with leg cramps and low back pain. Problems with corns, bunions and in-grown toenails are also aggravated.

Cardiovascular

Obesity is associated with hypertension. Blood pressure is further increased by a further weight gain and lowered by a weight reduction (Kopelman 1984). Weight gain is also associated with a rise in serum cholesterol and low density lipoprotein concentrations and a reduction in serum high density lipoprotein concentrations (Royal College of Physicians 1983). Obesity is also an important risk factor for the development of diabetes. Thus data from the Framingham study show that, among elderly men (65–94 years), there is an increased risk of cardiovascular disease with increasing relative weight (Kannel et al. 1986).

Respiratory

Severe obesity can cause hypoventilation during the day and episodes of apnoea during sleep (Kopelman 1984). The condition does not appear to be a particular problem in old age, but this may simply reflect under-investigation in the very old.

Metabolic

The complex relationship between obesity and carbohydrate metabolism is discussed in Chap. 4. There are increases in serum uric acid levels in obesity, but these are only associated with gout in men who are more than 130% overweight (Royal College of Physicians 1983).

Gastrointestinal

Although the majority of old people have a hiatus hernia, only a minority suffer from the symptoms of gastro-oesophageal reflux. Obese patients are at particular risk, however, in that their excess fat causes an increased gastro-oesophageal pressure gradient (Beauchamp 1983). Although such patients are often advised to lose weight, there have been no definitive trials to confirm benefit.

Obesity is associated with an increased risk of gallstones in women under 50, but has no association with these in older women or in men of any age.

Cancer

There is an actuarial association between obesity and cancer of the colon, rectum and prostate in men, and cancer of the breast, uterus and cervix in women (Low and Garfinkel 1979). It is unclear whether obesity increases the risk of cancer, or whether dietary factors cause both obesity and cancer (Editorial 1982).

Treatment

Treatment of obesity requires a high level of compliance and a considerable effort on the part of staff so that the therapeutic objectives should be clearly defined at the outset. In old age, improvement of mobility, a reduction in joint pain, or the relief of gastro-oesophageal reflux are important benefits. It is less likely that weight reduction will reduce the risk of heart disease, stroke, cholecystitis or cancer in the very old. Even if there are marginal changes those are unlikely to be important in a group with an extremely short life expectancy. Unfortunately, there has been little formal evaluation of strategies/or promoting weight loss in elderly individuals.

The only effective way of reducing fat mass is to decrease energy intake. An obvious, but widely ignored principle, is that weight loss will only occur if the energy intake is less than expenditure. This presents particular problems in disabled old people whose energy expenditure is often considerably less than 4 MJ per 24 h.

A reasonable approach is to start off with an energy intake of 4 MJ per day. If, over the course of 2 weeks, this has been ineffective, this should be reduced to 3.3 MJ.

While prescribing a diet, it is important to assess compliance. Even in hospital, it is often difficult to detect surreptitious raids on other patients' plates and lockers, or well-meaning but ill-conceived smuggling operations by friends and relatives. Eternal vigilance should be the watchword. At home, regular visits from a health visitor and attendance at a day hospital, particularly where an element of competition and reward is built into the regular weigh-ins, should prove helpful.

Many old people have fluid retention due to cardiac failure, drug treatment or local venous stasis, and fluctuations in this may confound attempts to monitor the effects of dietary restriction. A regular check should be made, therefore, for ankle and sacral oedema, jugular venous congestion, and evidence of pulmonary oedema.

Young and middle-aged people failing to respond to moderate dietary restriction have been successfully treated with a very low calorie diet (Wadden et al. 1983). This contains only 1.3 MJ consisting of around 45 g of protein and 30 g of glucose. It should be supplemented with vitamins and potassium (e.g. one tablet each of Orovite and Sando K daily). A fluid intake of between 1.5 and 2 l per day is important to avoid uraemia associated with tissue breakdown. The treatment has not yet been adequately evaluated in elderly patients, so that it should be only used with extreme caution in this group.

In the past, obesity has been treated by total fasting and there still are some advocates of this approach. There are disturbing reports, however, of patients on treatment developing ventricular fibrillation, small bowel infarction and lactic acidosis (Wadden et al. 1983). Again, many patients treated in this way fail to maintain their weight loss. A strong case could be made, therefore, for avoiding this approach in the elderly.

Many of the problems involved in achieving weight loss could be resolved if an effective anorectic agent was available. Most of those in current use have side-effects which are unacceptable in the elderly. An example is that fenfluramine can cause drowsiness, insomnia, depression and confusion and that these are particularly severe in old people.

Prevention

The general public should be advised that with increasing age and a decline in physical activity, an individual who does not reduce his calorie intake is likely to gain weight. Advice on maintaining a reasonable level of physical activity, and education on the energy content of different foodstuffs and the value of increased dietary fibre is useful. Venues for such education include pre-retirement courses, carer groups, day centres, day hospitals, senior citizens' clubs and luncheon clubs. Health visitors should also be encouraged to advise and monitor nutrient intakes when visiting old people at risk.

References

Bastow MD, Rifking J, Allison SR (1983) Benefits of supplementary tube feeding after fractured neck of femur: A randomised controlled trial. Br Med J 287: 1589–1592

Beauchamp G (1983) Gastro-oesophageal reflux and obesity. Surg Clin N Am 63: 869–876

Burr M, Phillips KM (1984) Anthropometric norms in the elderly. Br J Nutr 51: 165–169

Cheng AHR, Gomez A, Bergen JG et al. (1978) Comparative nitrogen balance study between young and aged adults using three levels of protein intake from a combination of wheat-soy-milk mixture. Am J Clin Nutr 31: 12–22

Durnin JVGA, Womersley J (1974) Body fat assessed from total body density and its estimation from skinfold thickness measurements on 481 men and women from 16–72 years. Br J Nutr 27: 537–542

Editorial (1982) Obesity: The cancer connection. Lancet 1: 1223–1224

Fentem PH, Jones PR, MacDonald IC et al. (1976) Changes in the body composition of elderly men following retirement from the steel industry. J Physiol 258: 29P–30P

Friedman PJ, Campbell AJ, Caradoc-Davies TH (1985a) Prognostic trial of a new diagnostic criterion for severe wasting malnutrition in the elderly. Age Ageing 14: 149–154

Friedman PJ, Campbell AJ, Caradoc-Davies TH (1985b) Hypoalbuminaemia in the elderly is due to disease not malnutrition. J Clin Exp Gerontol 7: 191–203

Garrow JS, Webster J (1985) Are pre-obese people energy thrifty? Lancet 1: 670–671

Jung RT (1984) Endocrinological aspects of obesity. Clin Endocrinol Metab 13: 597–612

Jung RT, Campbell RG, James WPT, Callingham BA (1982) Altered hypothalamic and sympathetic responses to hypoglycaemia in familial obesity. Lancet 1: 1043–1046

Kannel WB, Garrison RJ, Wilson PWF (1986) Obesity and nutrition in elderly diabetic persons. Am J Med 1986 80 (suppl 5A): 22–30

Kemm JR (1985) Vitamin deficiency in the elderly. Blackwell, London

Kopelman PG (1984) Clinical complications of obesity. Clin Endocrinol Metab 13: 613–614

Leach RE, Baumgard S, Broom J (1973) Obesity: Its relationship to osteoarthritis of the knee. Clin Orthop 93: 271–273

Lonergan ME, Milne JS, Maule MM, Williamson J (1975) A dietary survey of older people in Edinburgh. Br J Nutr 34: 517–527

Low EA, Garfinkel L (1979) Variations in mortality by weight among 750,000 men and women. J Chronic Dis 32: 563–576

MacLennan WJ (1983) Nutrition of the elderly in continuing care. In: Caird FI, Grimley Evans J (eds) Advanced geriatric medicine 3. Pitman, London, pp 9–20

MacLennan WJ (1985) Clinical assessment of nutritional status in the elderly. In: Kemm JR (ed) Vitamin deficiency in the elderly. Blackwell, London, pp 22–45

MacLennan WJ, Martin P, Mason BJ (1975) Energy intake, disability, disease and skinfold thickness in a long stay hospital. Gerontol Clin 17: 173–180

MacLennan WJ, Martin P, Mason BJ (1977) Protein intake and serum albumin levels in the elderly. Gerontology 23: 360–367

Masoro EJ (1984) Food restriction and the ageing process. J Am Geriatr Soc 32: 296–300

Montgomery RD, Heaney MR, Ross IN et al. (1978) The ageing gut: a study of intestinal absorption in relation to nutrition in the elderly. Q J Med 47: 197–211

Morgan DB, Newton HMV, Schorah CJ et al. (1986) Abnormal indices of nutrition in the elderly: a study of different clinical groups. Age Ageing 15: 65–76

Munsey WF (1981) Foot problems in the overweight. Postgrad Med 69: 33

Novak LP (1972) Ageing, total body potassium, fat-free mass, and cell mass in males and females between ages 18 and 65 years. J Gerontol 27: 437–443

Price HL, Gazzard BG, Dawson AM (1973) Steatorrhoea in the elderly. Br Med J 1: 1582–1584

Rennie MJ, Harrison R (1984) Effects of injury, disease and malnutrition on protein metabolism. Lancet 1: 323–325

Ross MH, Lustbader ED, Bras G (1985) Dietary habits and the prediction of life span of rats: A prospective test. Am J Clin Nutr 41: 1332–1344

Royal College of Physicians (1983) Obesity. J R Coll Physicians Lond 17: 5–65

Segal KR, Gatton B (1983) Thermic effects of food and exercise in lean and obese women. Metabolism 32: 581–589

Shephard RJ (1978) Physical activity and ageing. Croom Helm, London, pp 193–196
Shock NW (1955) Metabolism and age. J Chronic Dis 2: 687–703
Sidney KH, Shephard RJ (1977) Activity patterns of elderly men and women. J Gerontol 32: 25–32
Tomlinson BE, Irving D (1977) The numbers of limb motor neurones in the human lumbosacral cord throughout life. Neurol Sci 34: 213–219
Wadden TA, Stunkard AJ, Brownell KD (1983) Very low calorie diets: Their efficacy, safety and future. Ann Intern Med 99: 675–684
Webster SGP, Leeming JT (1975) Assessment of small bowel function in the elderly using a modified xylose tolerance test. Gut 16: 109–113
Webster SGP, Williamson EM, Gowland E (1977) A comparison of fat absorption in young and old subjects. Age Ageing 6: 113–117

11 Endocrine and Metabolic Effects of Drugs and Hormonal/Endocrine Manipulation of Non-endocrine Diseases

A wide range of drugs has an effect on the function of endocrine glands, may simulate or mask the effect of hormones, or may confound the interpretation of hormone assays. The problem is further complicated in the elderly by the fact that most patients present to the surgery, out-patient clinic or ward on at least one drug, and in many instances, a multiplicity of preparations.

Hormones are also often used as therapeutic agents in non-endocrine disorders, and it is important that the clinician is able to weigh the benefits against the adverse effects of such treatment. Ageing and co-existent disease frequently alter the balance of the equation, sometimes to the extent that treatment is no longer appropriate.

The present chapter addresses itself to these two issues.

Endocrine Effects of Drugs Commonly Used in Elderly Patients

Cardiac Glycosides

One of the side-effects of cardiac glycosides is gynaecomastia (Carlson 1980). An explanation for this is that glycosides have a high affinity for oestrogen receptors and thus act as oestrogen agonists (Rifka et al. 1978).

Diuretics

Both thiazide and "loop" diuretics have been implicated as indirect causes of impaired carbohydrate tolerance. In a trial of the combination of hydrochlorothiazide and triamterene (Dyazide) in elderly hypertensive patients, there was a significant rise in fasting blood glucose levels and deterioration in glucose tolerance tests over the course of 3 years (Amery et al. 1978) (Figs. 11.1 and 11.2).

The impairment in carbohydrate tolerance may be an indirect effect of hypokalaemia, a condition which reduces the secretion of insulin from pancreatic islet beta-cells. Certainly, in at least one study, correction of hypokalaemia resulted in a reduction of blood glucose levels (Heldeman et al. 1983).

Thiazide diuretics also effect changes in lipid metabolism reflected in a rise in plasma concentrations of triglyceride and low density lipoprotein cholesterol (Goldman et al. 1980; Grimm et al. 1981). These changes in glucose and lipid metabolism raise the question of whether treatment with thiazide diuretics increases the risk of cardiovascular disease (MacLennan 1984). Fortunately the balance of evidence is that the hypotensive effect of diuretics outweighs any adverse metabolic effect and, in general, reduces cardiovascular morbidity and mortality.

Diuretics commonly result in an increase in serum uric acid levels (Johnson and Mitch 1981). This is a direct consequence of diuretic efficacy in that it is a reduction in the plasma flow rate which causes volume depletion and an increase in solute resorption from the distal tubule.

Since both ageing and hypotension are associated with an elevation of serum uric acid levels, treatment of elderly hypertensive patients with diuretics poses

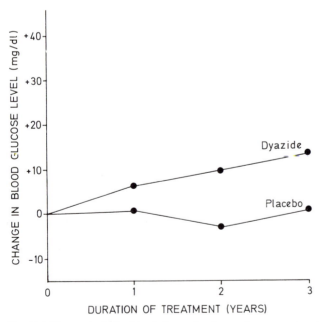

Fig. 11.1 Changes in fasting blood glucose levels over three years in patients on a diuretic and on a placebo. (After Amery et al. 1978.)

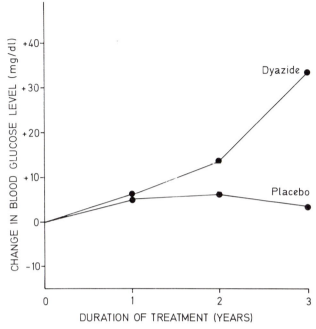

Fig. 11.2. Changes in blood glucose 2 h after 50 g oral glucose in patients on a diuretic and a placebo. (After Amery et al. 1978.)

particular problems. Fortunately, relatively few patients on diuretics with high serum uric acid levels develop gout (Dargie and Dollery 1975).

The effect of diuretics on electrolyte balance is reviewed in Chap. 9.

Beta-adrenergic Blocking Agents

All drugs in this group reduce the rate of hepatic gluconeogenesis. This is usually of little relevance, but under conditions of stress, such as fasting or severe physical exercise, it can lead to symptomatic hypoglycaemia (Holm et al. 1981).

The possibility of interactions between beta-blockers and hypoglycaemic agents has been extensively investigated. However, if patients are on a sulphonylurea, beta-blockers actually produce a marginal rise in blood glucose levels (Wright et al. 1979). Again, the incidence of hypoglycaemic coma in patients receiving insulin was no greater in those also treated with a beta-blocker (Barnett et al. 1980).

Oral Hypoglycaemic Agents

Chlorpropamide has frequently been incriminated as a cause of hyponatraemia (Tanay et al. 1981). It effects this by increasing the secretion of anti-diuretic hormone (ADH) from the posterior pituitary and increasing the sensitivity of the distal renal tubules to the same hormone. Tolbutamide also occasionally causes this syndrome, but glibenclamide has no effect on fluid balance, while acetohexamide, glipizide and tolazamide actually increase salt and water loss (Moses and Miller 1973). The latter may be the result of an increased glomerular filtration rate and impaired reabsorption of sodium from the proximal renal tubule.

Psychotropic Agents

Phenothiazines and butyrophenones, by virtue of their effect on neurotransmitters within the hypothalamus, have a wide range of metabolic effects. Increased secretion of ADH and prolactin may give rise to either hyponatraemia or gynaecomastia. The drugs may also cause sexual dysfunction, but this relates to changes in the autonomic nervous system rather than the pituitary. Patients are also at increased risk of developing hypothermia, but this also relates to changes in autonomic rather than metabolic function.

A more common side-effect is that of weight gain. The pathogenesis of this is unclear, but it is likely to relate to a change in appetite and intake, rather than in peripheral metabolism. It is encouraging to note that discontinuation of the offending drug is often followed by weight reduction.

Tricyclic Antidepressants

The metabolic side-effects of the tricyclic antidepressants are similar to those of the psychotropic agents, in that cases of inappropriate secretion of ADH and gynaecomastica occur from time to time. Weight gain is also common and relates both to relief of anorexia in depression and a change in taste perception (Nakra et al. 1977). Most of the more recently developed antidepressant compounds, maprotiline, doxepin, trazodone and mianserin for example, have similar effects on appetite and weight (Robinson 1984).

Drugs and Hormone Assays

Many drugs commonly used in old people interfere with the assay of serum concentrations of hormones and it is important that the clinician has a clear grasp of the effect of these on the results he obtains from his laboratory. Fortunately these problems are becoming less as more specific immunoassays for various hormones become available and particularly as the capacity increases to measure free rather than total hormone concentrations. Table 11.1 lists the effects which drugs have upon serum total thyroxine, total triiodothyronine and thyroid stimulating hormone levels and exemplifies the multiple levels at which drugs can interfere with evaluation of endocrine function.

Table 11.1. Effect of drugs commonly used in old age on serum thyroxine (T_4) and triiodothyronine (T_3) and thyroid stimulating hormone (TSH) (Werzel 1981)

Drug	Effect on T_4, T_3 or TSH	
Androgens	Decreased protein binding	
Salicylate	Transport binding competition	
Heparin	Transport binding competition	
Diazepam	Transport binding competition	
Sulphonylurea	Transport binding competition	
Fenclofenac	Transport binding competition	
Phenytoin	Enzyme induction	
Carbamazepine	Enzyme induction	
Phenobarbitone	Enzyme induction	
Propranolol	Inhibition of metabolism	
Co-trimoxazole	Thyroid inhibition	
Thiazides	Reduction in distribution volume	
Phenothiazines	Unknown	
Oestrogens	Increased protein binding	
Bromocriptine	Dopamine agonist	
L-Dopa	Dopamine precursor	alter
Metoclopramide	Dopamine antagonist	TSH
Cimetidine	Histamine anatagonist	responses

Effects of Drugs on Individual Endocrine Systems

The Thyroid

TSH secretion and the response of TSH to stimulation by TRH is enhanced by oestrogen therapy and theophylline and reduced by glucocorticoids and dopamine agents such as L-dopa and bromocriptine.

Hyperthyroidism may be seen during replacement therapy with excessive doses of thyroxine and is rarely due to a deliberate self-overdosage (thyrotoxicosis artefacta). The condition has always been commoner with thyroid extract than thyroxine and has also been reported following ingestion of hamburgers made from beef neck muscles contaminated with thyroid tissue (Hedberg et al. 1987). Again it may be induced by the administration of an iodide preparation (Jod-Basedow phenomenon). This is particularly common in patients who are iodine deficient or have a pre-existing simple goitre, but it may also occur in apparently normal individuals. Responsible medications have in the past included proprietary asthma remedies. Health products containing kelp are also iodine rich. Paradoxically iodide preparations can also induce hypothyroidism and goitre, either during short-term high dosage (Wolff-Chaikoff effect) or long-term low dosage.

Amiodarone presents particular problems as it may cause hyperthyroidism or hypothyroidism and it also is a potent inhibitor of the conversion of T_4 to T_3 and thus confuses the interpretation of thyroid function tests (Chap. 3).

A number of drugs other than the conventional antithyroid drugs can inhibit the utilisation of iodine and hence synthesis of thyroid hormones. They include chlorpropamide (Hunter et al. 1965), phenylbutazone, and acetozolamide. Aminoglutethimide also has this effect and it is recommended that supplementary thyroxine therapy be given with this drug (Hughes and Burley 1970).

In addition to amiodarone, propranolol has a modest effect on inhibiting the conversion of T_4 to T_3 resulting in a slight elevation of total T_4 and reduction in total T_3. This effect of adrenoreceptor blocking agents is shared to a lesser extent by some other beta-adrenoceptor antagonists (Feely and Peden 1984).

Many drugs can interfere with conventional tests for thyroid function by interfering with the binding of thyroid hormones to various plasma proteins (Table 11.1). An example is that oestrogens increase the concentration of TBG, thus elevating TT_4 and TT_3 levels. Androgens have the opposite effect. Tests such as the T_3 uptake, measuring residual binding sites and allowing the calculation of a free thyroxic index, overcome this to some extent. A number of drugs, including salicylates, fenclofenac and phenytoin effect binding of thyroid hormones to their binding sites. Again, enzyme inducing anticonvulsants reduce total and free T_4 concentrations and may also interfere with TSH secretion. This could compromise the use of a sensitive TSH assay as a first-line test of thyroid function in patients taking anticonvulsants, but the assay has effectively overcome the majority of the other in vitro drug-induced problems encountered with conventional thyroid function tests.

Adrenocortical Function

A number of enzymatic steps are involved in the synthesis of cortisol, and a number of drugs can inhibit one or more of these. The effect of metyrapone in blocking 11-beta-hydroxylase is used therapeutically in the management of Cushing's syndrome. Aminoglutethimide has a number of effects which include inhibition of the conversion of cholesterol to 5-pregnenolone, the conversion of androstenedione to oestrone, and increasing the metabolic clearance of dexamethasone. If aminoglutethimide is used therapeutically to inhibit steroid synthesis, hydrocortisone should be administered to prevent hypoadrenalism. Ketoconazole inhibits both steroidogenesis and cytochrome P450-dependent enzyme activity and interferes with steroid binding to receptors. Acute adrenal failure has also been reported in patients on oral anticoagulant therapy and the anaesthetic agent etomidate can also cause acute hypoadrenalism.

Drugs such as aminoglutethimide which inhibit cortisol synthesis may also interfere with aldosterone production.

A number of drugs interfere with the fluorometric assay of plasma and urine cortisol. The most common of these is spironolactone. Again prednisolone may interfere with certain radio-immunoassays for cortisol.

As noted above, hydrocortisone and the synthetic glucocorticoid drugs suppress the hypothalamic pituitary adrenal axis. Prolonged use of a large dose of glucocorticoid (>20–30 mg hydrocortisone or equivalent daily) can result in the suppression of hypothalamic-pituitary-adrenal axis for up to a year after its cessation.

Gonadal Function and Gynaecomastia

In addition to cardiac glycosides, other drugs commonly used in old people which cause gynaecomastia are spironolactone and cimetidine. They act by displacing dihydrotestosterone from its receptors to promote an anti-androgenic effect. Phenothiazines, benzodiazepines and tricyclic antidepressants may induce gynaecomastia by increasing the secretion of prolactin from the anterior pituitary. Isoniazid, ethionamide and griseofulvin also occasionally cause gynaecomastia. Oestrogens such as stilboestrol, used in the management of prostatic cancer cause gynaecomastia, testicular atrophy and proliferation and softening of scalp hair.

Diseases associated with gynaecomastia include chronic liver failure and thyrotoxicosis. Ageing itself has an influence on the prevalence of the condition, in that there is an increase from puberty onwards throughout adult life, later rising sharply to reach a peak in the seventh decade (Williams 1963). Changes in testicular function and in the peripheral metabolism of androgens have been suggested as explanations for this (Carlson 1980).

Vasopressin Secretion

The secretion of vasopressin is inhibited by alcohol, opioids and phenytoin so that all can promote diuretic effects. Demeclocycline and lithium inhibit the effects of vasopression on the kidney and thus may cause nephrogenic diabetes insipidus. A number of drugs have anti-diuretic effects. An example is that chlorpropamide enhances the renal effects of vasopressin thus causing hyponatraemia. In contrast, other sulphonylurea drugs including tolazamide and acetohexamide have a diuretic effect. Other drugs which cause hyponatraemia through water intoxication include carbamazepine, clofibrate, amitriptyline, monoamine oxidase inhibitors and the cytotoxic drugs vincristine, cyclophosphamide and carboplatin.

Carbohydrate Metabolism

Hyperglycaemia

The effect of thiazide diuretics on carbohydrate metabolism has already been described.

Other cardiovascular drugs including beta-adrenoceptor antagonists and calcium channel blockers modify insulin secretion. However, though these agents reduce insulin secretion in experimental situations, there is no evidence that chronic use interferes with glucose tolerance or carbohydrate metabolism. Profound insulin resistance and hyperglycaemia may also be precipitated by the use of intravenous salbutamol and adrenaline in intensive and coronary care situations.

Glucocortocoid drugs used in pharmacological doses cause insulin resistance. The onset of diabetes is often rapid but since insulin secretion is maintained ketosis is rare and hyperosmolar non-ketotic hyperglycaemic coma is more common. Synthetic oestrogens are also diabetogenic but the concentrated equine oestrogens used in hormone replacement therapy are the least likely of these drugs to have this effect.

Hypoglycaemia

Hypoglycaemia due to oral hypoglycaemic drugs is dealt with in Chap. 5.

Hypoglycaemia, whether due to sulphonylurea or insulin treatment, may be masked by concomitant treatment with beta-adrenoceptor blockers (Davidson et al. 1977). Tachycardia and tremor may be absent. A cardio-selective rather than a non-selective beta-blocker is of marginal advantage in this situation (Brass 1984).

Weight Gain

Weight gain is a potential side effect of a range of psychoactive drugs, particularly the anti-psychotic phenothiazines, the tricyclic antidepressants and lithium. It must be recognised that weight gain may be an index of treatment success in a depressed elderly patient. Antiserotonin drugs such as cyproheptadine and pizotifen cause weight gain, but are rarely indicated in elderly patients. Weight gain is also associated with glucocorticoid drugs or with the use of anabolic steroids in conditions such as osteoporosis.

Hormonal and Endocrine Manipulation of "Non-endocrine" Disease and its Adverse Effects

Corticosteroids

Corticosteroids may be indicated in a wide range of conditions affecting elderly patients, but their wide range of adverse effects means that their benefits are often outweighed by disadvantages. In some instances patients may progress to a dependency on corticosteroids for disorders such as asthma or rheumatoid arthritis. Corticosteroids, often in pharmacological rather than physiological doses, are indicated for disorders such as temporal arteritis, polymyalgia rheumatica, lymphoreticular or haemopoietic malignancy or cerebral oedema.

In general terms and depending on the necessary treatment regimen for the underlying problem, the aim should be to taper the steroid dose to the minimum essential to keep the condition satisfactorily controlled. If this dosage is equivalent to 7.5 mg of prednisolone or less (Table 11.2) then the chances of the patient becoming (or remaining) overtly cushingoid are significantly reduced (Table 11.3).

Table 11.2. Equivalent doses of natural and synthetic glucocorticoids

Hydrocortisone	30 mg
Cortisone acetate	37.5 mg
Prednisolone	6.0 mg
Triamcinolone	4.0 mg
Dexamethasone	0.75 mg
Betamethasone	0.75 mg

Table 11.3. Daily doses of prednisone required to control rheumatoid arthritis in patients aged over 60 (Lockie et al. 1983)

Dose (mg/day)	Number of patients
2.5	3
2.5–5	1
2.5–10	2
5.0	36
5.0–7.5	2
5.0–10.0	12
7.5	19
7.5–10.0	22
Total	97

The plethora of side-effects associated with corticosteroid therapy are listed in Table 11.4. The risk of these is compounded by the effects of ageing and multiple pathology so that old people on corticosteroids may present with one of a wide range of serious disorders which include depression, an acute confusional state, hyperglycaemic coma, congestive cardiac failure, extensive pressure sores, a stroke, haematemesis, immobility, a fractured proximal femur or lumbar vertebra, a pulmonary embolism, a perinephric or paracolic abscess, or miliary tuberculosis. Careful monitoring of the clinical state and fine tuning of dosage are essential if these problems are to be avoided.

Table 11.4. Side-effects of corticosteroid therapy

Hypertension	Leukocytosis
Confusion	Polycythemia
Mood changes	Thrombocytopenia
Reduced carbohydrate tolerance	Peptic ulceration
Salt and water retention	Obesity
Hypokalaemia	Osteoporosis
Increased capillary fragility	Avascular necrosis of bone
Hirsutism	Myopathy
Impaired wound healing	Infection, e.g. skin, lungs and kidneys
Pressure sores	Coronary thrombosis
Cataract	Deep vein thrombosis
Stroke	

A further risk is that long-term treatment with corticosteroids may result in suppression of pituitary-adrenal function (Christy 1973). The prevalence of this is dependent upon the criteria used to define it. Thus, of 19 patients on long-term corticosteroids for rheumatoid arthritis, only 32% had subnormal plasma cortisol responses to Synacthen, but another 26% had abnormalities relating to either the metyrapone, lysine-vasopressin or insulin-induced hypoglycaemia tests (Jasani et al. 1967).

If the clinical condition of the patient is stable, these abnormalities present no problems, but in a situation of stress, patients with subnormal pituitary-adrenal function often secrete inadequate amounts of cortisol (Jasani et al. 1968). Only a small proportion of patients with abnormal cortisol responses go on to present with clinical problems, but cases of corticosteroid-treated patients developing hypotension or dying suddenly during surgery or acute illness have been widely reported (Christy 1973).

These problems can be minimised if clinicians always aim at using the smallest dose of corticosteroids necessary to control a disorder. Regimens in which corticosteroids are given every second day reduce the risk of adrenal suppression, but may cause problems of compliance in the elderly. Treatment should be carried on for as short a period as possible, but withdrawal should be gradual both to allow recovery of pituitary-adrenal function and to minimise the risk of exacerbation of the original disease. On occasions, however, pituitary-adrenal dysfunction persists for as long as a year after steroid withdrawal.

If a patient on corticosteroids develops an intercurrent illness the dose of corticosteroid should be doubled, or increased to a maximum equivalent to 20 mg/day of prednisolone. If the patient cannot take oral medication then parenteral hydrocortisone should be substituted in an initial dose of 100 mg (Hall et al. 1980).

For surgery it is essential that parenteral hydrocortisone is given along with the pre-medication and continued for 24 h after minor surgery and for 72 h after major surgery. The dose is then tapered to the normal maintenance dosage. Even minor procedures such as endoscopy should be covered with a 100 mg dose of intramuscular hydrocortisone.

Problems arise in patients who have previously been treated with corticosteroids and who suffer major intercurrent stress or require surgery. The regimen already described should be given for surgery to any patient who has had corticosteroids in the previous 2 months. Indeed, patients who have apparently been successfully withdrawn from long-term steroid therapy may require cover for up to 2 years after cessation of treatment. Although steroid cover may be omitted if there is a normal cortisol response to insulin hypoglycaemia, the test is often contra-indicated in elderly patients so that it is easier and safer to provide routine cover.

Oestrogens and Anti-oestrogens

The use of oestrogens in post-menopausal problems and in osteoporosis has been described in Chaps 6 and 7, and in this section attention is given to their place in the management of carcinoma of the prostate and of the breast.

Carcinoma of Prostate

Stilboestrol has been used in the treatment of carcinoma of the prostate for over 30 years (Williams 1985). Initially, large doses were used but these caused a high mortality from cardiovascular disease, and it was found that small doses were equally effective. The principal action of stilboestrol in prostatic disease is to suppress the pituitary testicular axis, thus inhibiting testosterone secretion. A dose of 3 mg of stilboestrol daily is sufficient to produce testosterone levels equivalent to those of orchidectomy (Shearer et al. 1973). Stilboestrol is often given in combination with orchidectomy. The approach is based on a large review in 1950 which showed that oestrogens alone had little effect on long-term survival but that orchidectomy improved 5-year survival, and that orchidectomy with oestrogens produced a marginally better intermediate survival (Fig. 11.3) (Nesbitt and Baum 1950).

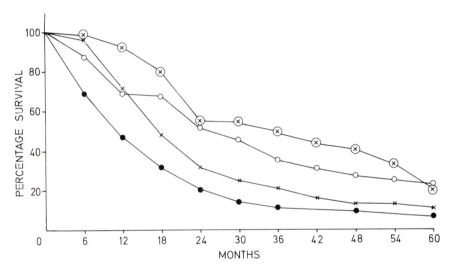

Fig. 11.3. Survival curves for patients with advanced carcinoma of the prostate who were untreated (*solid circles*), treated with oestrogens (*crosses*), treated with orchidectomy (*open circles*) or treated with orchidectomy and oestrogens (*crosses in open circles*). (After Nesbitt and Baum 1950.)

An alternative form of hormonal therapy is to use a luteinising hormone releasing hormone (LHRH) analogue (Williams 1985). This acts, after an initial short period of gonadotrophin stimulation, subsequently to cause down regulation of gonadotrophin LHRH receptors and to switch off secretion of luteinising hormone. This, in turn, eliminates the testicular secretion of androgens. The three agents in current use are buserelin, leuprolide and gosalerin. There also is a depot preparation of gosalerin which has the advantage of producing continuous rather than intermittent suppression of testosterone secretion.

These agents have not been in use for long enough to assess their effect on survival, but it is unlikely that this will be much different from that for oestrogen therapy or orchidectomy. Their main advantages may be that they do not increase the incidence of cardiovascular disease, and that they avoid the psychological trauma of orchidectomy.

Ketoconazole, an antifungal agent, inhibits steroidogenesis and interferes with the secretion of androgens from both gonads and adrenals (Williams 1985). It produces less effective suppression of testosterone levels than orchidectomy. However, combination treatment with a LHRH analogue results in the effective suppression of both gonadal and adrenal testosterone secretion. The clinical efficacy of this approach has not yet been established.

Carcinoma of Breast

A large proportion of patients with carcinoma of the breast have oestrogen-dependent tumours which are therefore amenable to hormonal therapy (Allegra 1983). Post-menopausal patients are more likely to have an oestrogen dependent lesion, but biopsy and biochemical analysis is necessary to establish this.

The drug most widely used in hormonal treatment is the anti-oestrogen agent tamoxifen. It is useful as an adjunct to surgery and, in a recent trial in women over 65 who had mastectomy for stage II carcinoma, 76% of those on tamoxifen were disease free at 4 years, compared with only 52% of those on placebo (Cummings et al. 1985). There was little difference in survival between the two groups, however. In extreme old age, the physical frailty and limited life expectancy means that surgery or radiotherapy is inappropriate. Tamoxifen given alone in this situation in a dose of 10 mg three times daily produced a reduction in tumour size in 68% of patients. It had little effect upon overall mortality, but since only 5 out of 14 deaths were related to the carcinoma, this is not surprising.

Progestagens are also used in breast cancer, but are more likely to be effective if the biopsy specimen contains progestagen receptors (Blumenschein 1983). They are normally reserved for patients who have failed to respond adequately to tamoxifen. The two oral regimens in current use are methylprogesterone acetate in a dose of 500 mg twice daily, and megestrol acetate in a dose of 80 mg twice daily.

Although aminoglutethimide was developed as an anticonvulsant, it also has the property of blocking the action of aromatase enzymes, substances essential for the conversion of androgens to oestrogens (Powles 1983). Trials in breast cancer have established that it is as effective as tamoxifen. It has a wide range of side-effects, however (Table 11.5). Although many of these are transient, lasting for less than a month, they can be troublesome, so aminoglutethimide is mainly reserved for patients with widespread metastases. Another limitation is that the drug suppresses adrenal as well as gonadal function, so corticosteroid supplements have to be given. As noted above, aminoglutethimide may also cause hypothyroidism.

The standard dose of aminoglutethimide is 250 mg three times daily. The smaller dose of 250 mg daily eliminates the need for corticosteroid supplements, but further experience is required on whether it achieves adequate tumour remission.

Investigations continue into the efficacy of combinations of hormone therapy (Stoll 1984). As yet, these have produced no convincing evidence of benefit over single drugs, but developing information on tumour cell metabolism and receptor sites may lead to more accurate strategies for this approach.

Table 11.5. Side-effects of aminoglutethimide (Powles 1983)

Side-effect	Percentage incidence
Lethargy	33
Nausea	15
Macular rash	23
Ataxia/muscle cramps	4
Blood dyscrasias	Rare

Hormones have also been used along with cytotoxic drugs, but discussion of this is outwith the remit of this book (Davidson and Lipman 1985).

Adverse Effects

Oestrogens

Large doses of oestrogens produce an increased mortality from cardiovascular causes in patients suffering from carcinoma of the prostate (Table 11.6) (Veterans Administration Co-operative Urological Research Group 1967). The risk is further increased if the patient already has cardiovascular disease before the start of treatment (Bennett et al. 1970). Reduction in the dose of oestrogen used reduces but does not eliminate the risk.

Table 11.6. Mortality from cardiovascular disease in patients with carcinoma of the prostate, treated or not treated with stilboesterol (Veterans Administration Co-operative Urological Research Group 1967)

Cause of death	Percentage incidence in patients	
	on oestrogen	not on oestrogen
Heart disease	15	9
Cerebrovascular disease	11	7

There is also concern about oestrogen replacement in post-menopausal women as a possible cause of cardiovascular disease and malignancy. In an attempt to minimise risks, it has been recommended that the dose of oestrogen should be small, that it should be given discontinuously and that it should be given along with a progestogen (Judd et al. 1981). Studies on small numbers of women over 10 years suggest that if these precautions are taken the risk of endometrial cancer is greatly reduced (Braunstein 1984). However, studies on larger numbers over a longer period are necessary to ensure that the technique completely eliminates the risk of cancer. The risk of postmenopausal women on oestrogens developing breast cancer has also been investigated, and no causal relationship has emerged. The criticism could again be made, however, that large enough numbers have not been studied for long enough (Morrow 1985).

When the influence of oestrogen therapy on non-neoplastic disease has been investigated no association with either myocardial infarction, stroke or thromboembolic disease has emerged (Braunstein 1984). Women on oestrogens, however, are twice to three times as likely to develop hypertension or gallbladder disease. Transdermal administration of oestrogens to hysterectomised women is now being advocated. It is claimed that this avoids the adverse effects on lipoproteins and clotting factors associated with the delivery of large oestrogen concentrations to the liver by oral preparations.

Tamoxifen

The side effects of tamoxifen are similar to those for oestrogens, but these are usually mild and rarely lead to withdrawal of therapy. Figures on the overall prevalence of side effects vary but are 10–20% for flushing, 5–15% for gastro-intestinal upset, and 5–10% for vaginal bleeding (Heel et al. 1978). An occasional problem is that tamoxifen causes acute progression of the underlying disease so that it exacerbates bone pain, causes hypercalcaemia, and causes inflammation of skin adjacent to tumour tissue (Plotkin et al. 1978). This represents an initial response to the drug as an agonist, which eventually subsides and is usually followed by tumour regression. The drug also causes transient thrombocytopenia in 5–15% of patients, but this usually settles when treatment is stopped. A few reported cases of pulmonary embolism occurring in patients on tamoxifen are more likely to have been the result of the underlying malignancy.

Anabolic Steroids

Though these drugs are not widely used in elderly patients at present, future research may establish a role for them in the treatment of cachexia or osteoporosis. It is important therefore that clinicians should be aware of their potential toxicity before proposing their more general use.

The most important side-effect is that of a high incidence of cholestatic jaundice. Salt and water retention also may be a problem, and may precipitate congestive cardiac failure, while changes in plasma lipoprotein fractions may increase the incidence of coronary artery disease. Cases of hepatic carcinoma have also been reported, but this only occurs after prolonged exposure. Vascular liver tumours have also been reported in patients taking anabolic steroids.

References

Allegra JC (1983) Rational approaches to the hormonal treatment of breast cancer. Semin Oncol 10 (suppl 4): 25–28

Amery A, Berthaux P, Bulpitt C et al. (1978) Glucose intolerance during diuretic therapy. Results of a trial by the European Working Party on Hypertension in the Elderly. Lancet 1: 681–683

Barnett AH, Leslie D, Watkins PJ (1980) Can insulin-treated diabetics be given beta-adrenergic blocking drugs? Br Med J 280: 976–978

Bennett AH, Dowd JB, Harrison JH (1970) Oestrogen and survival data in carcinoma of the prostate. Surg Gynecol Obstet 130. 505–508

Blumenschein GR (1983) The role of progestagens in the treatment of breast cancer. Semin Oncol 10 (suppl 4): 7–10

Brass EP (1984) Effects of antihypertensive drugs on endocrine function. Drugs 27: 447–458

Braunstein GD (1984) Opinion Pro: the benefits of oestrogen to postmenopausal women outweigh the risks of developing endometrial cancer. Canc J Clin 34: 210–219

Carlson HE (1980) Gynaecomastia. N Engl J Med 303: 795–799

Christy NP (1973) The clinical significance of pituitary-adrenal suppression by exogenous corticosteroids. J Chronic Dis 26: 261–263

Cummings FJ, Gray R, Davis TE et al. (1985) Adjuvant tamoxifen treatment of elderly women with stage II breast cancer. Ann Intern Med 103: 324–329

Dargie HJ, Dollery CT (1975) Adverse reactions to diuretics. In: Dukes MNG (ed) Meyler's side effects of drugs, vol. 8. Excerpta Medica, pp 483–501

Davidson NE, Lipman ME (1985) Combined therapy in advanced breast cancer. Eur J Clin Oncol 21: 1123–1126

Davidson NM, Corrall RJM, Shaw TRD et al. (1977) Observations in man of hypoglycaemia during selective and non-selective beta-blockade. Scot Med J 22: 69–72

Feely J, Peden NR (1984) Use of β-adrenoceptor blocking drugs in hyperthyroidism. Drugs 27: 425–446

Goldman AI, Steele BW, Schnafer HE et al. (1980) Serum lipoprotein level during chlorthalidone therapy. JAMA 244: 1691–1695

Grimm RH, Leon AS, Hunninghake DB et al. (1981) Effects of thiazide diuretics on plasma lipids and lipoproteins in mildy hypertensive patients. Ann Intern Med 94: 7–11

Hall R, Anderson J, Smart GA, Besser M (1980) The fundamentals of clinical endocrinology, 3rd edn. Pitman Medical, Tunbridge Wells

Hedberg CW, Fishbein DB, Jansen RS et al. (1987) An outbreak of thyrotoxicosis caused by the consumption of bovine thyroid gland in ground beef. N Engl J Med 316: 993–998

Heel RC, Brogden RN, Speight TM, Avery GS (1978) Tamoxifen: a review of its pharmacological properties and therapeutic use in the treatment of breast cancer. Drugs 16: 1–24

Heldeman JH, Elahi D, Anderson DK et al. (1983) Prevention of the glucose intolerance of thiazide diuretics by maintenance of body potassium. Diabetes 32: 106–111

Holm G, Herlitz J, Smith U (1981) Severe hypoglycaemia during physical exercise and treatment with beta-blockers. Br Med J 282: 1360

Hughes SWM, Burley DM (1970) Aminoglutethimide: side effect turned to therapeutic advantage. Postgrad Med J 46: 409–411

Hunter RB, Wells MV, Skipper EW (1965) Hypothyroidism in diabetics treated with sulphonylureas. Lancet 2: 449–451

Jasani MK, Boyle JA, Greig WR et al. (1967) Corticosteroid-induced suppression of the hypothalamo-pituitary-adrenal axis: observations on patients given oral corticosteroids for rheumatoid arthritis. Q J Med 36: 261–276

Jasani MK, Freeman PA, Boyle JA et al. (1968) Studies on the rise in plasma 11-hydroxycorticosteroids (11-OHCS) in corticosteroid-treated patients with rheumatoid arthritis during surgery: correlation with the functional integrity of the hypothalamo-pituitary-adrenal axis. Q J Med 37: 407–421

Johnson MW, Mitch WE (1981) Opinion Pro: the risks of asymptomatic hyperuricaemia and the use of uricaemic diuretics. Drugs 21: 220–225

Judd HL, Clearly RE, Creasman WT et al. (1981) Oestrogen replacement therapy. Obstet Gynecol 58: 267–275

Lockie LM, Gomez E, Smith DM (1983) Low dose adreno-corticosteroids in the management of elderly patients with rheumatoid arthritis: selected examples and summary of efficacy in the long-term treatment of 97 patients. Semin Arthr Rheum 12: 373–382

MacLennan WJ (1984) Use and abuse of diuretics. In: Evans JG, Caird FI (eds) Advanced geriatric medicine. 4. Pitman, London, pp 127–141

Morrow CP (1985) Opinion Con: The benefits of oestrogen to the menopausal woman outweigh the risks of developing endometrial cancer. Canc J Clin 34: 220–231

Moses AM, Miller M (1973) Diuretic action of three sulphonylurea drugs. Ann Intern Med 78: 541–544

Nakra BR, Rutland P, Varma S, Gaind R (1977) Amitriptyline and weight gain: a biochemical and endocrinological study. Curr Med Res Opin 4: 602–606

Nesbitt RM, Baum WC (1950) Endocrine control of prostatic carcinoma: Clinical and statistical survey of 1,118 cases. JAMA 143: 1317–1320

Plotkin D, Lechner JJ, Jung WE et al. (1978) Tamoxifen: place in advanced breast cancer. JAMA 240: 2644–2646

Powles TJ (1983) The role of aromatase inhibitors in breast cancer. Semin Oncol 10 (suppl 4): 20–24

Rifka SM, Pita JC, Vigersky RA et al. (1978) Interaction of digitalis and spironolactone with human sex steroid receptors. J Clin Endocrinol Metab 46: 338–344

Robinson DS (1984) Adverse reactions, toxicities, and drug interactions of newer antidepressants: anticholinergic, sedative, and other side effects. Psychopharmacol Bull 20: 280–290

Shearer RJ, Hendry WJ, Sommerville IF, Ferguson JD (1973) Plasma testosterone: an accurate monitor of hormone treatment in prostatic cancer. Br J Urol 45: 668–677

Stoll BA (1984) Combination endocrine therapy in breast cancer. Eur J Cancer 21: 413–416

Tanay A, Fireman Z, Yust I, Abramov AL (1981) Chlorpropamide-induced syndrome of inappropriate antidiuretic hormone secretion. J Am Geriatr Soc 29: 334–336

Veterans Administration Co-operative Urological Research Group (1967) Treatment and survival of patients with cancer of the prostate. Surg Gynecol Obstet 124: 1011–1017

Werzel KW (1981) Pharmacological interference with in vitro tests of thyroid function. Metabolism 30: 717–732

Williams MJ (1963) Gynaecomastia. Its incidence, recognition and host characterisation in 447 autopsy cases. Am J Med 34: 103–112

Williams G (1985) Endocrine treatment of prostatic cancer. J R Soc Med 78: 797–799

Wright AD, Barber SG, Kendall MJ, Poole PH (1979) Beta-adrenoceptor blocking drugs and blood sugar control in diabetes mellitus. Br Med J 1: 159–161

12 Investigation of Endocrine Disease

The purpose of this chapter is to provide a brief description of tests of clinical relevance to the investigation of endocrine disorders in the elderly. Information is also provided on ranges of values found in healthy old people. These, however, have often been obtained from highly selected populations and there are wide variations in laboratory techniques used. Discussion with local chemical pathologists is therefore essential to the effective interpretation of results. Since our book is intended mainly for clinicians, no attempt has been made to describe the details of assay techniques. Again, no mention has been made of techniques which, though useful as research tools, have little influence on the management of individual patients.

Thyroid Disease

Conventional TSH radio-immunoassay lacks sensitivity in the lower part of the normal range and cannot reliably distinguish a low normal value in a euthyroid individual from a suppressed value in a hyperthyroid patient. A number of highly sensitive TSH assays have recently been developed, utilising labelled monoclonal antibodies and immunoradiometric (IRMA) chemiluminescent or enzymatic assays. The sensitive TSH assays are claimed to distinguish between normal TSH values (above 0.2 mU/l) in euthyroidism and suppressed TSH values in hyperthyroidism. There is a strong correlation between plasma TSH levels using sensitive methodology and the TSH increment during TRH testing.

With the advent of the sensitive TSH assay, new strategies for testing thyroid function have been suggested (Caldwell et al. 1985). The basal serum TSH level using sensitive methodology can reliably distinguish between primary hyperthyroidism, the euthyroid state and primary hypothyroidism. Basal TSH concentration measured by sensitive methodology is always suppressed when the TSH increment on TRH testing is less than 1 mU/l. It can therefore replace TRH testing in the exclusion of hyperthyroidism (Seth et al. 1984).

The last few years have also seen the development of commercial immunoassay techniques (both isotopic and non-isotopic) for the direct measurement of free T_4 and free T_3 in serum. Many laboratories now measure free T_4 in preference to total T_4, or the derived free thyroxine index. These assays, on the whole, function satisfactorily and may be more sensitive than the total T_4 as an index of hyperthyroidism. They permit accurate diagnosis of patients with abnormalities of thyroxine binding globulin (TBG), although problems remain in their interpretation in patients with other abnormalities of thyroid hormone-binding proteins and in non-thyroidal illness (Seth and Beckett 1985). Increasingly, the role of either free or total thyroid hormone assays is to confirm the thyroid status suggested by a sensitive TSH assay, the thyroid hormones being elevated when the TSH is suppressed in hyperthyroidism, and reduced when the TSH is elevated in primary hypothyroidism. Full evaluation of sensitive TSH and free thyroid hormone assays in elderly patients is awaited.

Healthy, young and old subjects have similar reference ranges for the serum total T_4 (65 – 145 nmol/l) (Caplan et al. 1981). The normal range for serum total T_3 reported in young adults as 1.3–2.6 nmol/l falls in men and women over the age of 65 to 0.9–1.7 nmol/l (Caplan et al. 1981).

Until recently, the response of serum TSH levels to an intravenous bolus of TRH was the gold standard investigation for confirming the presence of hyperthyroidism, but since the basal TSH by sensitive methodology correlates well with the TSH increment during TRH testing, the TRH test is now mainly used in the investigation of hypothalamic pituitary disease. Normally 200 µg TRH is given intravenously and blood samples taken for TSH assay before, and 20 and 60 min after injection. A TSH rise of greater than 1 mU/l rules out hyperthyroidism. In young adults, a basal value of less than 5 mU/l normally rises by at least 3 mU/l after 20 min and falls thereafter. The response is considered exaggerated if the 20 min TSH value is above 25 mU/l in men and post-menopausal women. Opinions differ on whether age has any effect on the results of TRH tests (Ordene et al. 1983; Harman et al. 1984). Any changes are minor, however, so that diagnostic criteria applied in youth are probably also appropriate in old age. TSH responses to TRH injection may be reduced in seriously ill patients.

Measurement of serum thyroidal auto-antibodies, particularly thyroglobulin and thyroid microsomal antibodies, may be helpful in defining the aetiology of hyperthyroidism and goitre in elderly patients (Tunbridge et al. 1977). The role of antibodies against TSH receptors in the pathogenesis of hyperthyroid Graves' disease has been discussed in the chapter on thyroid disease. Such receptor antibody studies are not at present widely used in routine clinical practice.

The role of thyroid scintigraphy, ultrasonography and needle biopsy in the evaluation of nodular disease of the thyroid has been dealt with in the chapter on thyroid disease.

Diabetes Mellitus

The diagnosis of diabetes mellitus is made on the basis of a random venous plasma glucose (hereafter blood glucose) concentration of over 11.1 mmol/l (Chap. 4).

As has already been emphasised, the diagnostic criteria for the diagnosis are the same in the elderly as in the young adults.

A glucose tolerance test need only be performed on patients in whom the random blood glucose level gives an equivocal result (7.8–11.0 mmol/l). As a preliminary to the test a 150 g carbohydrate diet should be given for at least three days. The patient is fasted on the morning of the test and then given a 75 g oral dose of glucose with water (250–350 ml over 5 min). The critical blood glucose levels are those at fasting and at 2 h. Intermediate values may be rarely necessary in asymptomatic individuals.

Measurement of plasma insulin levels and C-peptide levels may be useful in research studies but the response of the pancreas to a glucose load is too variable for an insulin profile to be of any great value in the diagnosis of diabetes, or in the distinction between insulin-dependent and non-insulin-dependent forms (Keen and Ng Tang Fui 1982). An exception to this is that, in late onset patients, lean patients with low peak insulin responses more frequently require insulin therapy (Lyons et al. 1984).

In all individuals, glucose becomes linked by a non-enzymatic chemical reaction to the terminal valine residue of the haemoglobin B chain. The process involves a reversible reaction to form an intermediate aldimine base, which can then undergo an irreversible Amadori re-arrangement to form a stable ketoamine. The resulting glycosylated haemoglobin defined as HbA_{1C} is one of four minor variant haemoglobin A_1 molecules. This reaction occurs throughout the life-cycle of the red cell and the higher the ambient glucose concentrations, the higher is the resulting haemoglobin A_{1C} (or total HbA_1) concentration. The glycosylated haemoglobin concentration is therefore an index of glycaemic control over the preceding 2–3 months (Ashby et al. 1985).

In an insulin-dependent patient a glycosylated haemoglobin assay performed every 4–6 months can be used to assess diabetic control, and is a valuable check on the reliability of home blood glucose monitoring. Glycosylated haemoglobin levels are less necessary in non-insulin-dependent diabetes, where glycaemic control as estimated by HbA_1 correlates well with both the fasting and random blood glucose levels checked at an out-patient clinic (Paisey et al. 1980).

Gonadal Function

Although ageing and disease have major effects on gonadal function, detailed information on this is rarely of much value in the management of individual patients. Endocrinological assessment may be indicated in some patients presenting with gynaecomastia, or erectile impotence, or where hypothalamic pituitary dysfunction is considered. The issue of serum testosterone concentrations in healthy old men and in those with acute or chronic illness has been addressed in Chap. 1. Further information on hypothalamo-pituitary-testicular axis function may be obtained from basal gonadotrophin levels and their response to intravenous stimulation with LHRH. Both concentrations and responses are low in patients with hypothalamic pituitary dysfunction and high in patients with primary gonadal disorders. It has also recently been recognised that apparently non-functional pituitary tumours frequently synthesise and secrete gonadotrophins or their A and B subunits. Healthy elderly men have elevated oestradiol concentrations and the imbalance between oestradiol and testosterone in this age group may result in gynaecomastia. A prolactinoma may be associated with hypogonadism, and older patients with this disorder tend to have very high basal prolactin concentrations.

Elderly women are, by definition, post-menopausal and have high basal gonadotrophin concentrations. Indeed, in an otherwise well elderly female, low gonadotrophin levels are a sensitive pointer to hypopituitarism.

Bone Disease

Serum calcium, inorganic phosphate and alkaline phosphatase concentrations are extremely useful in the identification of metabolic bone disease. Although the reference range of serum calcium levels in young and old are the same at 2.20–2.60 mmol/l, many sick old people have a low serum albumin concentration. It is essential that a correction be made for the resultant reduced calcium-binding capacity of the serum. The "corrected" serum calcium concentration can be calculated by adding or subtracting 0.02 mmol/l of calcium for every 1 g/l of albumin below or above a concentration of 40 g/l.

Whereas the range of serum organic phosphate levels in younger subjects is 0.80–1.55 mmol/l, those for elderly men and women are 0.61–1.25 and 0.76–1.42 mmol/l respectively. The upper limit of normal for the serum alkaline phosphatase is one of 100 iU in young adults compared with that of 140 iU in the elderly. There is speculation as to whether the change is the result of undetected Paget's disease in the latter group.

Calcidiol (25-hydroxyvitamin D) is the main circulating metabolite of vitamin D, and its status has been extensively investigated in the elderly (MacLennan et al. 1979). Although many old people with low levels of calcidiol do not have osteomalacia, a serum calcidiol level of less than 15 nmol/l associated with a low serum calcium or elevated serum alkaline phosphatase level increases the likelihood of the diagnosis often eliminating the need for a bone biopsy (Burns and Paterson 1985).

Calcitriol (1,25-dihydroxycholecalciferol) is the only vitamin D metabolite to have a direct effect on calcium homeostasis, and is intimately associated with PTH secretion, but serum levels of it are subject to such large and rapid fluctuations that its assay is of little diagnostic value (Mawer 1980).

Since immunoassay techniques for identifying the amino terminal, carboxy terminal, or midmolecular components of PTH have become available, assays of the hormone have been much more useful in confirming the diagnosis of hyperparathyroidism (Lindall et al. 1983). There is a rise in both serum concentrations of amino-terminal and mid-molecular antigens in the elderly (Peterson et al. 1983;

Marcus et al. 1984). In healthy old people, the upper limit for the assay is 50% greater than in those under 50. This difference is probably the result of a decline in renal function associated with age. In patients admitted to a geriatric unit, the upper limit was increased by around 500%, and the main reason for this was a renal response to vitamin D deficiency and a low serum calcidiol concentration.

In healthy old people, the simplest way of coping with the problem would be to reset limits of normal for the range of PTH levels. If the elderly patient is sick or housebound, however, serum calcidiol levels should be checked to exclude the likelihood that the high PTH level is secondary to vitamin D deficiency.

Studies on the urinary excretion of calcium and phosphate are of limited value in old people because of the difficulty of obtaining accurately timed collections. A partial solution to the problem is to measure the ratio of the calcium concentration to that of the creatinine in an untimed specimen of urine (Bulusu et al. 1970). The test is occasionally useful in defining the cause of hypercalcaemia.

Hypothalamic Pituitary Disease

Evaluation of the Hypothalamic-Pituitary-Adrenal Axis

Suspected ACTH Deficiency

Fortunately this is an uncommon problem in elderly patients since there are potential problems with the conventional stimulation tests. Initially a 09.00 h basal plasma cortisol concentration should be measured and a short Synacthen test performed.

The procedure is to give 250 µg of tetracosactrin (Synacthen) IM between 0800 and 1000 h withdrawing blood at time zero and at 30 and 60 min after injection. Normally the basal cortisol level is 170 to 690 nmol/l with post-injection levels being at least 550 nmol/l, and the peak minus basal increment being greater than 308 nmol/l. In a patient with other evidence of hypopituitarism, an abnormal basal cortisol or deficient response to Synacthen supports the diagnosis.

The conventional stimulation test of ACTH reserve is the insulin-induced hypoglycaemia or tolerance test (ITT). This is contra-indicated in patients with ischaemic heart disease or epilepsy and arguably also in patients with cerebrovascular disease and indeed in all patients over the age of 65 years (Wand and Ney 1985). If the test is considered to be essential, then the basal cortisol and the cortisol response to Synacthen should have been tested and have been established as normal.

In the ITT, insulin is given intravenously. The usual dose is 0.1 units/kg, although larger doses are necessary in insulin-resultant states such as acromegaly. Blood is taken prior to insulin injection and at 30, 45, 60 and 90 min thereafter. Glucose and a variety of hormones may be measured during the ITT. These include cortisol, ACTH (if available), growth hormone and prolactin. The blood glucose should fall to less than or equal to 2.2 mmol/l, or less than 50% of the basal value. The test must be supervised by a medically qualified person. Ninety minutes after the injection the patient may be fed but he should be kept under observation for a further 2 h.

If symptoms of hypoglycaemia are severe, the hypoglycaemia may be reversed by oral or intravenous glucose without the need to terminate sampling. In this case intravenous hydrocortisone should be administered at the end of the test.

An alternative to the ITT is to stimulate ACTH and growth hormone secretion with glucagon. This is useful in investigating suspected hypopituitarism in elderly patients (Belchetz 1984a, b). The procedure is to fast the patient and give 1 mg of glucagon subcutaneously. Blood is taken initially and at 90, 120, 150, 180, 210 and 240 min after injection. This should give a peak plasma cortisol level of greater than 550 nmol/l.

Synthetic corticotrophin releasing factor (CRF) has recently become more freely available, and has increasingly been used to stimulate the pituitary adrenal axis (Wand and Ney 1985). This approach is likely to present fewer risks than the ITT and may thus be more generally applicable to the elderly. Indeed a combined pituitary stimulation test using four releasing hormones (CRF, GHRH, LHRH and TRH) administered rapidly and sequentially has been developed (Sheldon et al. 1985) but it is still under investigation and has not yet been validated in old people.

Metyrapone can be used to evaluate ACTH reserve. This is a competitive inhibitor of 11-betahydroxylase which blocks the conversion of 11-deoxycortisol (11-DOC) to cortisol. It is given orally in a dose of 30 mg/kg at 24.00 h, and blood is sampled at 09.00 h for the serum 11-DOC level. In both young and old patients this should exceed 7 μg/dl. Metyrapone stimulation tests of ACTH reserve utilising urinary 17-hydroxicorticosteroid measurements are time consuming and unreliable. The test occasionally induces symptoms of acute adrenal insufficiency and should therefore only be performed under medical supervision in hospital.

A further and safer approach is to carry out a prolonged ACTH stimulation test in patients with an abnormal short Synacthen test. In this, 1 mg of tetracosactrin depot is given intramuscularly daily for 3 days, and the short Synacthen test is then repeated on day 4. If there is ACTH deficiency the peak cortisol should be greater than 700 nmol/l but if the problem is one of primary adrenocortical failure the cortisol should be less than 280 nmol/l.

Suspected Primary Adrenocortical Insufficiency (Addison's Disease)

The standard screening test is the short Synacthen test as described above. Elderly subjects show similar responses to those of younger subjects. Primary adrenocortical failure may be differentiated from secondary failure on clinical grounds (e.g. heavy pigmentation). Useful laboratory tests are the long ACTH stimulation test, and the plasma ACTH level. The latter is usually greater than 300 ng/l morning and evening in Addison's disease, but low or undetectable in a patient with adrenocortical insufficiency secondary to hypopituitarism.

Hypercortisolism (Cushing's Syndrome)

This diagnosis is often considered in obese, plethoric, hypertensive, diabetic patients, but is rarely sustained. It is useful to screen such patients for hypercortisolism using an overnight dexamethasone suppression test and the urinary free cortisol, both of which can be done on an out-patient basis.

In the overnight dexamethasone suppression test, a 1 mg oral dose of dexamethasone is given at 24.00 h and cortisol levels are measured between 08.00 and 10.00 h the following morning. The plasma cortisol level should fall to less than 150 nmol/l. False positive tests may occur in obesity, depression, or alcoholism (alcoholic pseudo-Cushing's syndrome).

The urinary free cortisol is usually measured in a 24-h urine collection, but may also be assessed as a cortisol : creatinine ratio in an early morning urine specimen. A normal 24 h urine free cortisol is less than 300 nmol. The test is usually normal in the obese patient, but may give false positives in alcoholism and depression.

Though false negative results are rare, they can occur if Cushing's disease has a cyclical pattern. This means that if the clinical suspicion is high, further evaluation should be made. The following tests are used for more detailed evaluation:

1. Loss of diurnal plasma cortisol variability. The 2200 hour cortisol is usually less than 275 nmol/l (but may be higher on the first night of admission to hospital), while the 0900-h cortisol should be less than 720 nmol/l.
2. Failure of cortisol to fall during formal low dose dexamethasone suppression. 0.5 mg of dexamethasone is given orally six hourly for 48 h. The 0900 plasma cortisol drawn on day 3 should be less than 180 nmol/l. The 24-h urinary 17 hydroxicorticosteroid secretion should fall to less than 4 mg/24 h during this test. Patients with depression may also have abnormal results.

The distinction between a depressed patient and one with Cushing's disease can be made by performing an ITT (insulin dose 0.3 units/kg). Patients with depression show a rise in their plasma cortisol level while patients with true Cushing's syndrome do not.

Once the diagnosis of hypercortisolism has been confirmed, the differential diagnosis is usually made using a high dose dexamethasone suppression test. In this test, dexamethasone 2 mg orally is given six-hourly for 48 h. This should suppress plasma cortisol or urinary 17 hydroxycorticosteroids by greater than 50% in patients with pituitary-dependent Cushing's disease. It does not have this effect in patients with adrenal adenoma or carcinoma. Patients with ectopic ACTH production from tumours usually have very high ACTH levels and only 10% show a fall of cortisol on high doses of dexamethasone (Howlett et al. 1985).

Patients with bronchial carcinoid as the source of the ACTH may have biochemical tests indistinguishable from those of patients with true pituitary-dependent Cushing's disease. They may also show a brisk rise in plasma ACTH plasma, 11-DOC or urinary steroids during a metyrapone test.

Stimulation tests using CRF are of little value in that exaggerated ACTH responses have been reported in patients with both pituitary dependent Cushing's disease and ectopic ACTH production.

The measurement of plasma ACTH levels during a dexamethasone suppression test is useful in patients with adrenal adenoma or carcinoma who have suppressed basal ACTH levels. In such patients, the adrenal lesion can be delineated with CT scanning. Indeed, CT scanning of the adrenals is increasingly advocated as the next step in investigation once hypercortisolism is confirmed, as this technique will reliably identify most adrenal tumours obviating the need for further complex biochemical investigation. Occasionally, venous sampling for ACTH may be necessary to determine an unusual site of ACTH production. This can be followed by CT scanning to delineate the lesion more accurately.

In cases of pituitary-dependent Cushing's disease, X-rays of the pituitary fossa are usually normal. Most patients have microadenomas and high resolution CT scanning of the pituitary fossa is required to identify these.

Prolactin

Basal serum prolactin levels are usually less than 400 mU/l but are variable and particularly prone to rise in response to stress, including venesection. In the differential diagnosis of hyperprolactinaemia, once drug administration and the presence of co-existent disease such as renal failure have been excluded, there is occasionally difficulty in deciding whether a patient is harbouring a pituitary microadenoma secreting prolactin. In such patients, repeated basal prolactin measurements are helpful, and the higher the basal prolactin, the more likely is the presence of a tumour. It has been suggested that loss of diurnal prolactin variation (higher in sleep), an impaired rise in response to TRH and metoclopromide support a diagnosis of prolactinoma. In patients with prolactinoma the production level is often >3000 mU/l. In patients with other pituitary tumours which cause pressure on the pituitary stalk, reducing the portal blood flow, prolactin levels are often modestly elevated because of removal of hypothalamic dopamine inhibition from the normal prolactin secreting cells.

If prolactin levels support a diagnosis of prolactinoma, then X-rays of the pituitary fossa are particularly likely to show enlargement in male patients, while high resolution CT scanning may reveal a microadenoma or, with appropriate contrast enhancement, reveal the extent of a macroadenoma.

Growth Hormone

Hypersecretion of growth hormone from a pituitary tumour is determined by measuring the effect of a glucose load on growth hormone levels. A standard glucose tolerance test is performed and in addition to samples for blood glucose, samples for plasma growth hormone are taken. Growth hormone levels should fall to below 2 mU/l in both young and elderly subjects. In acromegalic subjects paradoxical rises in growth hormone are often seen in response to both oral glucose and stimulation with TRH, LHRH and L-Dopa.

In an elderly patient growth hormone deficiency is likely to occur in the context of hypopituitarism. As has been noted earlier, conventional testing by ITT is generally contra-indicated in elderly patients. Growth hormone deficiency can be demonstrated with the glucagon stimulation test described previously. The recent identification of growth-hormone-releasing hormone (GHRH) and the development of this compound for stimulation testing has provided a safe and specific test for growth hormone deficiency although growth hormone responses to GHRH are affected by ageing (Chap. 1).

Adrenal Mineralocortocoid Function

Since primary hyperaldosteronism is rare and the definitive investigations time consuming, expensive and potentially invasive, and the case for surgical management in an elderly patient tendentious, it is important that simple screening tests should be used to separate out the bulk of the elderly patients who do not have the condition (Ferriss et al. 1981).

Spontaneous hypokalaemia of less than 3.0 nmol/l should be investigated particularly if this is associated with poorly controlled hypertension. However, around 10% of patients with primary hyperaldosteronism (PHA) have serum potassium values persistently above 3.7 nmol/l. In most instances, hypokalaemia is associated with diuretic therapy and thus should not be investigated. Ideally the same potassium concentration should be estimated on samples taken with the patient still supine after an overnight sleep. An erect posture results in a marginal rise in plasma potassium concentrations.

Once drug-induced hypokalaemia has been excluded, the main differential diagnosis of PHA is that of secondary hyperaldosteronism usually associated with renal or renovascular disease. The hallmark of PHA is a high (or high normal) supine plasma aldosterone level in the presence of a low or low normal supine plasma renin level. This differentiates patients with PHA from those with secondary hyperaldosteronism.

Confirmation of PHA can be made by a saline suppression test. This may be hazardous in patients with known cardiac disease. If after infusion of 2 l normal saline over four hours, the plasma aldosterone level has not been suppressed to less than 276 pmol/l, the diagnosis of primary hyperaldosteronism is probable and more definitive investigations, both to distinguish between an adrenal adenoma and idiopathic adrenal hyperplasia and to localise an adenoma, should be performed. These are described in detail elsewhere (Drury 1985; Peden 1986).

Adrenal Medullary Function

Investigation of adrenal medullary function is rarely indicated in elderly patients and should only be undertaken if patients have suspected phaeochromocytoma or idiopathic postural hypotension. The simplest approach is to measure the urinary excretion of catecholamine metabolites as vanillylmandelic acid (VMA). Normal values vary with individual laboratories but are less than 50 mmol per 24 h. Certain foodstuffs and drugs can interfere with the assay. They include coffee, tea, vanilla, bananas, chocolate, ice cream, nalidixic acid, methyldopa, imipramine, mono-amine oxidase inhibitors and reserpine. The urinary total metadrenaline excretion is more precise and gives fewer false negatives. Urinary catecholamine assays are more difficult to perform but give a positive pick-up rate for phaeochromocytoma in excess of 90%.

Assay of plasma catecholamines by radio-immunoassay methods represents the most specific test of sympatho-medullary function. Samples should be drawn from patients who have been supine for 30 min and should be transported in ice. The plasma should then be separated and stored at −20°C. Clonidine suppression testing with measurement of plasma catecholamines has come additional value in confirming the diagnosis of phaeochromocytoma, in that this interferes with the normal suppression of catecholamine levels by clonidine.

Once clinical and biochemical criteria have established the diagnosis of phaeo-chromocytoma, definitive radiology should be used to localise the tumour. A chest X-ray should be obtained to identify an intrathoracic tumour. At other sites CT scanning is the definitive method for tumour localisation. Such procedures as angiography and venous sampling should only be done in a patient whose clinical condition is stable, and in whom alpha-adrenergic, and if necessary, beta-adren-ergic blockade has been established.

Fluid and Electrolyte Balance

Renal Function

Age-related changes in renal function affect the interpretation of a variety of tests of metabolic function. It is important, therefore, that the clinician should be able to assess renal function in old age, and appreciate the constraints which age changes place upon investigations more appropriate for younger patients.

Both blood urea and serum creatinine levels provide only a limited amount of information about renal function in the elderly. Factors such as fluid intake, treat-ment with diurctics, protein intake, body weight and muscle mass also have a major effect on them. A nomogram has been used for calculating the glomerular filtration rate from the blood urea, serum creatinine and body weight (Denham et al. 1975). However, the technique is very inaccurate in that estimates of glomeru-lar filtration range between 50% and 200% of the real value.

The standard test for glomerular function is the creatinine clearance test. There are problems, however, in obtaining accurate 24-h collections of urine from frail elderly patients, and in this situation there may be advantages in using a radio-isotope test which does not require a timed sample of urine. An example is that radioactive-chromium-labelled EDTA can be injected intravenously and its clear-ance estimated from blood samples taken at 2, 3 and 4 h (Chantler et al. 1969). Estimates of the glomerular filtration rate calculated from this correlate well with those estimated by using inulin.

The ability of the kidney to concentrate urine can also have a major effect on fluid and electrolyte balance. This is tested by injecting 5 units of pitressin subcutaneously (Morrison 1979). This is given at 08.30 h and osmolality of the urine assessed on a sample collected between 14.30 and 16.30 h. In healthy young adults, the osmolality should exceed 750 mosmol/kg and elderly subjects are likely to produce less concentrated specimens.

Disorders of Vasopressin–Anti-diuretic Hormone (ADH) Secretion

Vasopressin deficiency manifesting as cranial diabetes insipidus occasionally occurs in old age, but a more common problem is the syndrome of inappropriate anti-diuretic hormone secretion (SIADH), described in Chap. 9. In the patient presenting with hyponatraemia, SIADH is suggested by low serum osmolality and inappropriately elevated urine osmolality. Clinical estimation of the extracellular fluid volume in such patients suggests that they are not dehydrated and, in addition, measurement of the urinary sodium usually reveals this to be greater than 40 mmol/l in SIADH. This is the result of a secondary natriuresis possibly due to atrial natriuretic peptide secretion in response to volume expansion. Measurement of vasopressin levels is available in a few specialised centres but is usually only indicated for research purposes. In patients with suspected cranial diabetes insipidus, a normal serum and urine osmolality from first morning specimens excludes the diagnosis. If this is not the case, a water deprivation test may be performed. The test is carefully monitored, particularly in elderly subjects, so that the patient does not drink water surreptitiously and is regularly weighed. The test is terminated when the urine osmolality has reached its maximum concentration, that is when two consecutive specimens show a variation in osmolality of less than 10% with at least a 2% drop in body weight. At this point serum sodium, serum osmolality and urine osmolality are measured (and ideally the serum vasopressin concentration). The patient is then given 5 units aqueous pitressin subcutaneously or desmopressin (DDAVP) 2 µg intramuscularly and the effect of this on urine osmolality noted.

Patients with both primary polydipsia and diabetes insipidus produce washout changes in their renal medullary gradient. Continued drinking in association with this washout prevents some patients with partial cranial diabetes insipidus from concentrating their urine osmolality by a further 10% above the plateau level of urine osmolality in the water deprivation test (the value normally taken to demonstrate a response to the exogenously administered pitressin). Such a disorder can be difficult to distinguish from patients with primary polydipsia. An additional problem is that some patients with nephrogenic diabetes insipidus may have some rise in urine osmolality after administration of pitressin.

Plasma vasopressin levels can be helpful in that they are very high in patients with nephrogenic diabetes insipidus. A sensitive vasopressin assay, if available, differentiates the low levels of vasopressin characteristic of patients with partial cranial diabetes insipidus, from the complete absence of vasopressin in complete diabetes insipidus.

The investigation of polyuria and the individual tests has been well reviewed (Baylis and Gill 1984).

Nutritional Status

The use of triceps skinfold thickness to assess fat deposition, and of the arm muscle area to assess muscle mass, are described in Chap. 10. In measuring skinfold thickness, Harpenden calipers should be used. The technique involves pinching the skin and subcutaneous tissues with the thumb and forefinger and then positioning the calipers and taking a reading when the needle on the attached dial slows down. Three readings are taken, and the mean of these is recorded. Considerable skill is required in standardising the technique, so that, if several individuals are involved in taking recordings, it is important to make inter-observer comparisons from time to time. Tables 12.1 and 12.2 give the 5th and 95th percentiles for these indices for men and women of various ages from 65 years and upwards (Burr and Phillips 1984).

Despite doubts as to the extent to which the serum albumin concentration is a reflection of protein intake, it is at least an index of nitrogen balance. Table 12.3 gives 95% confidence limits for this in elderly men and women.

Table 12.1. Percentiles for triceps skinfold thickness (Burr and Phillips 1984)

Age (years)	Percentiles for men (mm)		Percentiles for women (mm)	
	5th	95th	5th	95th
40–69	3.6	18.2	9.9	32.5
70–74	3.7	17.3	8.2	31.1
75–79	3.6	13.6	7.5	28.4
80–84	3.5	12.3	6.2	26.2
85+	3.4	12.2	6.0	21.8

Table 12.1. Percentiles for arm muscle area (Burr and Phillips 1984)

Age (years)	Percentiles for men (mm^2)		Percentiles for women (mm^2)	
	5th	95th	5th	95th
60–69	187	275	163	245
70–74	184	270	158	244
75–79	182	260	161	239
80–84	176	254	151	233
85+	172	244	141	223

Table 12.3. Ninety-five per cent confidence limits for serum albumin levels (Committee on Medical Aspects of Food Policy 1979)

Age (years)	95% confidence limits in men (g/l)		95% confidence limits in women (g/l)	
65–79	36.3	50.5	36.9	49.9
80+	33.3	50.9	35.8	49.6

References

Ashby JP, Deacon AC, Frier BM (1985) Glycosylated haemoglobin in Part 1: Measurement and clinical interpretation. Diabetic Med 2: 83–85

Baylis PH, Gill GV (1984) Investigation of polyuria. Clin Endocrinol Metab 13: 295–310

Belchetz PE (1984a) Idiopathic hypopituitarism in the elderly. Br Med J 291: 247–248

Belchetz PE (1984b) Anterior pituitary hormone problems. In: Belchetz PE (ed) Management of pituitary disease. Chapman and Hall, London, p 510

Bulusu L, Hodkinson A, Nordin BEC, Peacock M (1970) Urinary excretion of calcium and creatinine in relation to age and body weight in normal subjects and patients with renal calculus. Clin Sci 38: 601–612

Burns J, Paterson CR (1985) Single dose vitamin D treatment for osteomalacia in the elderly. Br Med J 290: 281–282

Burr ML, Phillips KM (1984) Anthropometric norms in the elderly. Br J Nutr 51: 165–169

Caldwell G, Kellett A, Gow SM, Beckett GJ, Sweeting VM, Seth J, Toft AD (1985) A new strategy for thyroid function testing. Lancet 1: 117–119

Caplan RH, Wickus G, Glasser JE et al. (1981) Serum concentrations of the iodothyronines in elderly subjects: decreased triiodothyronine (T_3) and free T_3 index. J Am Geriatr Soc 29: 19–24

Chantler C, Garnett ES, Parsons V, Veall N (1969) Glomerular filtration rate measurement in man by the single injection method using ^{51}Cr-EDTA. Clin Sci Mol Med 37: 169–180

Committee on Medical Aspects of Food Policy (1979) Nutrition and health in old age. Report on Health and Social Subjects No. 16, DHSS, HMSO

Denham MJ, Hodkinson HM, Fisher M (1975) Glomerular filtration rate in sick elderly inpatients. Age Ageing 2: 32–36

Drury PL (1985) Disorders of mineralocorticoid activity. Clin Endocrinol Metab 14: 175–202

Ferriss JB, Brown JJ, Fraser R et al. (1981) Primary hyperaldosteronism. Clin Endocrinol Metab 10: 419–452

Harman SM, Wehmann RE, Blackman MR (1984) Pituitary-thyroid hormone economy in healthy ageing men: basal indices of thyroid function and thyrotrophin responses to constant infusion of thyrotrophin releasing hormone. J Clin Endocrinol Metab 58: 320–326

Howlett TA, Rees LH, Besser GM (1985) Cushing's syndrome. Clin Endocrinol Metab 14: 911–946

Keen H, Ng Tang Fui S (1982) The definition and classification of diabetes mellitus. Clin Endocrinol Metab 11: 279–305

Lindall AW, Elting J, Ellis J, Ross BA (1983) Estimation of biologically active intact parathyroid hormone in normal and hyperparathyroid sera by sequential N-terminal immunoextraction and midregion immunoassay. J Clin Endocrinol Metab 57: 1007–1014

Lyons TJ, Kennedy L, Atkinson AB et al. (1984) Predicting the need for insulin therapy in late onset (40–69 years) diabetes mellitus. Diabetic Med 1: 105–108

MacLennan WJ, Hamilton JC, Timothy JI (1979) 25-hydroxyvitamin D concentrations in old people living at home. J Clin Exp Gerontol 1: 210–215

Marcus R, Madvig P, Young G (1984) Age-related changes in parathyroid hormone and parathyroid hormone action in normal humans. J Clin Endocrinol Metab 58: 223–230

Mawer EB (1980) Clinical implications of measurements of circulating vitamin D metabolites. Clin Endocrinol Metab 9: 63–79

Morrison RBI (1979) Urinalysis and assessment of renal function. In: Black D, Jones NF (eds) Renal disease. Blackwell, London, pp 305–327

Ordene KW, Pan C, Barzel US, Surks MI (1983) Variable thyrotrophin response to thyrotrophin-releasing hormone after small decreases in plasma thyroid hormone concentrations in patients of advanced age. Metabolism 32: 881–888

Paisey RB, MacFarlane DG, Sheriff RJ et al. (1980) The relationship between blood glycosylated haemoglobin and hormone capillary blood glucose levels in diabetics. Diabetologia 19: 31–34

Peden NR (1986) Primary hyperaldosteronism. Hosp Update 12: 865–880

Peterson MM, Briggs RS, Ashby MA et al. (1983) Parathyroid hormone and 25-hydroxyvitamin D concentrations in sick and normal elderly people. Br Med J 287: 521–523

Seth J, Beckett G (1985) Diagnosis of hyperthyroidism: the newer biochemical tests. Clin Endocrinol Metab 14: 373–396

Seth J, Kellett HA, Caldwell G, Sweeting VM, Beckett GJ, Gow SM, Toft AD (1984) A sensitive immunoradiometric assay for serum thyroid stimulating hormone. A replacement for the thyrotrophin releasing hormone test? Br Med J 289: 1334–1336

Sheldon WR, De Bold CR, Evans WS et al. (1985) Rapid sequential intravenous administration of four hypothalamic releasing hormones as a combined anterior pituitary function test in normal subjects. J Clin Endocrinol Metab 60: 623–630

Tunbridge WMG, Evered DC, Hall R et al. (1977) The spectrum of thyroid disease in a community: the Whickham survey. Clin Endocrinol 7: 481–493

Wand GS, Ney RL (1985) Disorders of the hypothalamic-pituitary-adrenal axis. Clin Endocrinol Metab 14: 33–54

Subject Index